Bhagavad Gita

Copyright © Yoga Satsanga Ashram 2021

Written by
Yogachariya Jnandev Giri

Editor
Yogacharini Deepika Saini

Proofread by
Dharma Simmons, Dharmananda Yoga and Mindfulness

ISBN 978-1-914485-03-9

First Published October 2021

Designed, Printed & Published by Design Marque

Printed in Great Britain by www.designmarque.co.uk

With Gratitude

I sincerely dedicate this Bhagavad Gita contemplative work to My Guru Ammaji Meenakshi Devi Bhavanani and my Parents.

Yogacharya Jnandev Giri (Surender Saini)

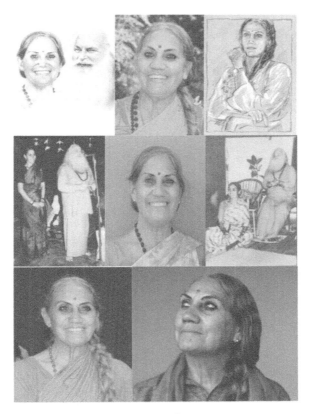

Ammaji, Yogacharini Smt Meenakshi Devi Bhavanani's 70th Jayanthi Celebrations 2013. www.icyer.com

Panchamahabhuta
Content List

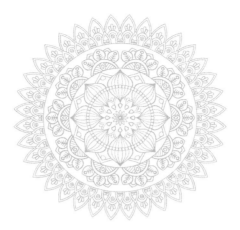

Bhagavad Gita
Introduction

The **Bhagavad Gita** (Sanskrit: Bhagavad Gītā) is an ancient Sanskrit text comprising of 700 verses from the Mahabharata (Bhishma Parva chapters 25 – 42). Krishna, as the speaker, counsellor and guide of the Bhagavad Gita is referred to as Bhagavan (the divine or supreme one). Each verse using the range and style of Sanskrit meter (chandas) with expressions and metaphors, comparing one with others - like brave as a lion - are written in a very poetic style. The title 'Gita' translates to "the Song of the Divine One". The Bhagavad Gita is revered as the most sacred literature by the majority of Hindus, and especially followers of Krishna and Yoga. In general speech it is known as The Gita.

The age of the Bhagavad Gita has been debated for decades by Indian and Western historians. The majority of western historians assume a date between 500 and 50 BCE. Theories based on archeoastronomy calculations from events of the Mahabharata conclude that the events of the Gita may have happened around 5561BC. The traditional date reflecting the beliefs of many devotional Hindus places the text in the 4th millennium BC.

There is, however, considerable debate on whether the Bhagavad Gita was written at the same time as the Mahabharata. Based on the differences in the poetic styles and supposed external influences such as Patanjali's Yoga Sutra, some scholars have suggested that the Bhagavad Gita was added to the Mahabharata at a later date.

This scripture or text is a dialogue between Lord Krishna and Arjuna (one of the five Pandva Brothers) taking place on the battlefield of Kurukshetra as part of the epic Mahabharat. The dialogue happens just before the battle was about to begin and finds Arjuna confused, deluded and in a moral dilemma as to whether he should fight against his brothers, uncles, teachers and relatives or not. Lord Krishna counsels Arjuna to follow his Dharma, to fulfil his duties as a warrior and take part in the war.

Arjuna's heart was filled with doubt and so he refused to fight. He turns to his charioteer and guide, Lord Krishna (an incarnation of Lord Vishnu), for guidance. Krishna explains to Arjuna about his duties as a warrior and Prince and elaborates on a number of different Yogic and Vedantic philosophies, with examples and analogies. This refers to the Gita as a guide to Hindu Dasrshana or viewpoints on life, karma, dharma and various paths of self-realisation. During the discourse, Krishna reveals his identity as the Supreme Being Himself (Bhagavan), blessing Arjuna with an awe-inspiring glimpse of His divine absolute form.

Swami Vivekananda, the follower of Sri Ramakrishna, was known for his commentaries on the four Yogas - Bhakti, Jnana, Karma and Raja Yoga - from his knowledge and understanding of the Bhagavad Gita. Swami Sivananda advises the aspiring Yogi to read verses from the Bhagavad Gita every day. Paramahamsa Yogananda, writer of the famous "Autobiography of a Yogi", viewed the Bhagavad Gita as one of the world's most divine scriptures. Swamiji Dr Gitananda Giriji has written a very easy and interesting poetic translation of the Bhagavad Gita and places it as a Key Yoga Scripture along with the Yoga Sutras of Patanjali.

The Bhagavad Gita describes the mind as turbulent and obstinate and as 'The Charioteer of the Body': the five horses represent the five senses (tongue, eyes, nose, ears and skin). The driver is the intelligence, or Buddhi, and the passenger is the spirit or soul.

Krishna counsels Arjuna that the soul is both eternal and immortal. Any 'death' only involves the physical body, but not the soul, as the soul is eternal. The soul changes its body like we change our clothes. Krishna summarises each of the Yogas through eighteen chapters. There are four kinds of Yoga - Raja Yoga, Bhakti Yoga, Karma Yoga, and Jnana Yoga.

Krishna elaborates in detail on Bhakti Yoga, the path of devotion, Karma Yoga, the path of skillful and desireless action, Dhyana Yoga or path of meditation, and Jnana Yoga or path of knowledge.

The Bhagavad Gita explains that one can only attain enlightenment by freeing themselves from the Ego and then realisation of the Truth or Reality of the immortal Self (the soul or Atman). Through detachment from the material sense of ego or I-ness, the Yogi, or follower of one of the paths of Yoga, is able to transcend from ego, attachment and illusory mortality and attains the realm of the Supreme Bliss or Joy: Satchidananda.

To demonstrate his divine nature, Lord Krishna grants Arjuna the boon of cosmic vision and allows him to perceive his 'Universal Form'. He reveals that he is fundamentally both the ultimate essence of Being in the universe, and also its material body, called the Vishvarupa.

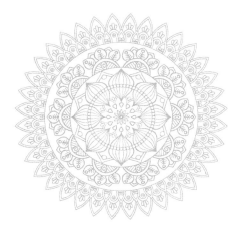

18 Paravas of Mahabharata

Mahabharata is one of the greatest written Hindu epics of all times. The historical events are composed in over 100000 slokas, or over 200000 verses - each sloka is a set of verses. It is written by Maharishi Veda Vyasa, in Sanskrit. Consisting of about 1.8 million words, the Mahabharata is almost 4 times longer than the Ramayana. The Mahabharata, meaning the great battle, narrates the epic Kurukshetra war and the fates of the Pandava and Kaurava princes. It is cantered around the central theme of Dharma, and contains values for virtuous or righteous living. The Mahabharata has been written in eighteen books, known as Parvas. The eighteen parvas are:

Parva	Title	Sub-Parvas	Contents
1	Adi Parva (The Book of the Beginning)	1-19	How the Mahabharata came to be narrated by Sauti to the assembled rishis at Naimisharanya. The recital of the Mahabharata at the sarpasattra of Janamejaya by Vaishampayana at Taksaśilā. The history of the Bharata clan is detailed and the parva also traces the history of the Bhrigu race. The birth and early life of the Kuru princesor dynasty is detailed. (adi means first, or prior to)
2	Sabha Parva (The Book of the Assembly Hall)	20-28	Maya Danava erects the palace and court (sabha), at Indraprastha. Life at the court, Yudhishthira's Rajasuya Yajna, the game of dice, and the eventual exile of the Pandavas are all detailed in this Parva.
3	Vana Parva also Aranyaka-parva, Aran-ya-parva (The Book of the Forest)	29-44	The events of the Padava princes' twelve years of exile in the forest (aranya) is detailed in this Parva.
4	Virata Parva (The Book of Virata)	45-48	This Parva details the 1-year the Padavas spent in disguise at the court of Virata.
5	Udyoga Parva (The Book of the Effort)	49-59	Preparations for war and efforts to bring about peace between the Kurus and the Pandavas which eventually fail (udyoga means effort or work).
6	Bhishma Parva (The Book of Bhishma)	60-64	The first part of the great battle, with Bhishma as commander for the Kauravas and his fall on the bed of arrows. This Parva contains teachings of the Bhagavad Gita.
7	Drona Parva (The Book of Drona)	65-72	The battle continues, with Drona as a commander. This is the major part regarding stories and events of the battle. Most of the great warriors on both sides are dead by the end of this Parva.
8	Karna Parva (The Book of Karna)	73	The events of the battle during which Karna was commander.

9	Shalya Parva (The Book of Shalya)	74-77	The last day of the battle, with Shalya as commander. Also told in detail is the pilgrimage of Balarama to the fords of the river Saraswati and the fight between Bhima and Duryodhana which ends the war, since Bhima kills Duryodhana by smashing him on the thighs with a mace.
10	Sauptika Parva (The Book of the Sleeping Warriors)	78-80	Ashvathama, Kripa and Kritavarma kill the remaining Pandava army while they sleep. Only 7 warriors remain on the Pandava side and 3 on the Kaurava side.
11	Stri Parva (The Book of the Women)	81-85	Gandhari, Kunti and the women (stri) of the Kurus and Pandavas lament the dead.
12	Shanti Parva (The Book of Peace)	86-88	The crowning of Yudhisthira as king of Hastinapura, and instructions from Bhishma for the newly appointed king on society, economics and politics. This is the longest book of the Mahabharata (shanti means peace).
13	Anushasana Parva (The Book of the Instructions)	89-90	The final instructions (anushasana) from Bhishma.
14	Ashvamedhika Parva (The Book of the Horse Sacrifice)	91-92	The royal ceremony of the Ashvamedha (Horse sacrifice) conducted by Yudhisthira to unite Bharatvarsh and establish peace.
15	Ashramavasika Parva (The Book of the Hermitage)	93-95	The eventual deaths of Dhritarashtra, Gandhari and Kunti in a forest fire when they are living in a hermitage in the Himalayas. Vidura predeceases them and Sanjaya, on Dhritarashtra's bidding, goes to live in the higher Himalayas.
16	Mausala Parva (The Book of the Clubs)	96	The infighting between the Yadavas with maces (mausala) and the eventual destruction of the Yadavas.

17	Mahaprasthanika Parva (The Book of the Great Journey)	97	The great journey of Yudhisthira and his brothers across the whole country and finally their ascent of the great Himalayas where each Pandava falls except for Yudhisthira.
18	Svargarohana Parva (The Book of the Ascent to Heaven)	98	Yudhisthira's final test and the return of the Pandavas to the spiritual world (svarga).
khila	Harivamsa Parva (The Book of the Genealogy of Hari)	99-100	Life of Krishna which is not covered in the 18 parvas of the Mahabharata.

Where exactly is Bhagavad Gita written?

Ramayana and Mahabharata are two of the greatest epics written in poetic Sanskrit and are known as Itihasas which means 'thus happened'. They contain the historic stories of ancient Kings who lived and ruled in India thousands of years ago. Both these historical epics contain many stories interwoven with teachings of dharma.

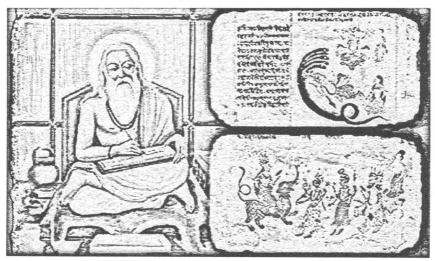

The Bhagavad Gita is part of the great Hindu epic Mahabharata, written by Maharishi Veda Vyasa.

The Bhagavad Gita appears in the middle of the story of Mahabharata. According to some historians, the period of Mahabharata was around 2500 to 5500 BCE. It is in the form of a dialogue between Lord Krishna, an incarnation of Lord Vishnu, and the great warrior Arjuna, just before the epic war at Kurukshetra was to begin.

In which language was the Bhagavad Gita written?

All ancient scriptures of Hinduism (Shruti and Smiritis) inclusive of the Mahabharata were written in Sanskrit language, also known as Devanagri (the language of gods).

Is the Bhagavad Gita part of the Vedas, the Hindu scriptures?

No. The Bhagavad Gita is not part of the four Vedas. Vedas are the original and ancient source scriptures of Hinduism and they are known as Shruti (as heard). They are believed to have originated directly from God and so no specific authors are attributed to Vedas.

The Bhagavad Gita is one of the very important and widely read and acclaimed scriptures of Hindu spiritual wisdom and comes under the group of scriptures known as Smritis (as remembered). Smritis are written by specific authors and so came much later than the Vedas but they have their connection to the Vedas. Smritis are meant to explain, elaborate and interpret Vedic wisdom.

Who was the author of the Bhagavad Gita?

The Bhagavad Gita is a discourse of spiritual wisdom given by Lord Krishna to his friend and disciple Arjuna. The Bhagavad Gita is written as part of the Mahabharata and hence Maharishi Vyasa was indeed the author or recorder of the Bhagavad Gita.

Why is it Known as the Bhagavad Gita?

Bhagavad Gita means 'song of the God'. Here it means teachings by Divine or Supreme Consciousness Parmatman. Vyasa compiled the Mahabharata and the Gita in poetry form.

What was the cause of the epic war Mahabharat?

The Kurukshetra or Mahabharata war is still considered as a war of dharma (righteousness) against adharma (anarchy or injustice). The five Pandavas (sons of Pandu and Kunti, Yudhisthira, Bheema, Arjuna, Nakul and Sahadev) who were on the side of dharma were fighting against 100 Kauravas (sons of Dhritarashtra and Gandhari). Dhritarashtra was a blind king of the Kuru clan ruling the Kuru kingdom headed by his eldest son Duryodhana.

Pandu and Dhritarashtra were brothers and hence the Pandavas and Kauravas were cousins. The Mahabharata narrates a historical epic story leading to the war within a family.

The Pandavas fought to get back their rightful share of their land and kingdom, confiscated by Kauravas by treachery during a game of dice. The Kauravas tried to humiliate the Pandavas by disrobing Pandava's wife Panchali (Draupadi) after their defeat in the game.

The Kauravas sent the Pandavas to the forest and put in place some stringent conditions if they ever wanted to get back their land. The Pandavas fulfilled these conditions successfully, but still the Kauravas did not want to return their land and rule. A war between them became inevitable.

In this epic war at Kurukshetra, all the kings who ruled so many countries across the length and breadth of Bharata Varsha (Indian Subcontinent) took part, siding with either the Kauravas or Pandavas according to what they believed was right. Arjuna was the brother of Yudhisthira and was the most valiant warrior and a great archer. He was virtually the hero of the Pandavas.

Krishna (an Incarnation or Avatar of Lord Vishnu) was a great warrior and a kingmaker at the kingdom of Yadavas and was a distant cousin of the Pandavas. Krishna and Arjuna were best friends.

Well before the war was about to begin, Krishna did his best to avoid the war. He himself went as a Shantidoot (diplomatic peace messenger) and used all his diplomatic skills to mediate peace between Pandavas and Kauravas. He offered several compromises and concessions to the Kauravas from the Pandavas' side so that a war between brothers could be avoided. But due to Duridhana's arrogance, greed and confidence that he could kill the Padavas with help of the greatest of warriors like Bhisma, Dronachariya, Karna and many more, this massive war became totally unavoidable. The pandavas too were very determined to fight and annihilate the adharmic Kauravas and re-establish a kingdom based on dharma, with Krishna's divine, moral support at their side.

How Krishna Becomes Arjuna's Charioteer

Before the war, the Pandvas and Kauravas went out to seek help from all the Kings and warriors. Both Arjuna and Duryodhana wanted Krishna's support for their respective group and came to seek his help.

Duryodhana arrived before Arjuna at Krishna's palace while he was sleeping and took the seat by his head while Arjuna arrived second but took the seat by his feet. When Krishna woke up, he saw Arjuna before Duryodhana and asked Arjuna first what he wished for.

Krishna offered his entire army to one side and his physical and moral support without taking up arms to another side. He asked them both to choose what they preferred. Arjuna was the first to decide and he chose Krishna's support only. Duryodhana, unaware of Krishna's divinity and due to his own ignorance and greed was happy to receive the huge army of Krishna for his side. Arjuna asked Krishna to be his charioteer and guide.

Arjuna's Confusion and Delusion over whether to Participate in War

When the Pandavas and Kauravas were growing up, they played together and studied together. However the Kauravas did not like Pandavas and created lots of troubles for them and even tried to kill them several times.

Both the groups received the love and care of their mighty Pitamaha (Great Grandfather) Bhishma. Bhishma was the elder brother of their grandfathers; he was indeed the real heir of Kuru kingdom, but he had renounced his rights, based on an oath to benefit his father.

Both groups studied together and learned archery and other war skills from Gurus Dronacharya and Kripacharya. The Acharyas were particularly fond of Arjuna who was extremely skilled in archery.

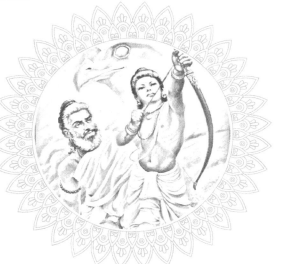

Despite the undercurrent of enmity, the Pandavas had maintained some sort of cordiality and entertained their brothers well when they became owners of their own kingdom with Indraprastha as its capital.

Arjuna did possess a soft heart for his erstwhile relatives deep down in his heart and also lots of respect and love for his Acharyas. Unfortunately, the mighty grandfather Bhishma and his teachers Kripacharya and Dronacharya (and his son Ashwathama) sided with the Kauravas in the war on account of their loyalty to the Kuru Kingdom. Some other kings who were their relatives were also at the side of the Kauravas.

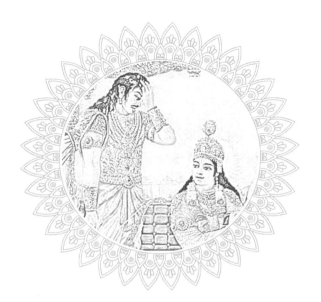

Just before the war began, Arjuna wanted to take a close look at the people of both sides ganged up against each other in the war. Krishna took the chariot to the front, facing the opponents.

It was then Arjuna suddenly became very weak-hearted. He saw his own cousins, his most respected Great Grandfather Bhishma, his masters Kripa and Drona standing up in the war against his side.

With Lord Krishna on his side, he was sure that the war would be won by the Pandavas, but all the people who were his relatives and beloved teachers, now standing in front of him, would be killed. He was caught by the emotions of attachment and he felt very bad about such an outcome.
At this point the whole war looked meaningless to Arjuna. He was gripped by a sudden inexplicable feeling of confusion, even delusion, and felt like renouncing all his cherished desires, duties and his ancestral rights to the Kingdom and escape everything and live as a hermit or Sadhu.

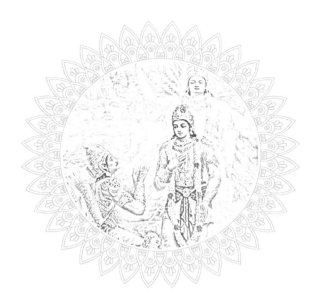

Krishna, Arjuna's charioteer became his counsellor

Arjuna was a very close friend of Krishna, so close as to call him 'Yadava' while Krishna called him Bandhu (brother) and Sakha (friend). Arjuna was also aware of the fact that Krishna is a divine incarnation of Vishnu, a personification of divine universal wisdom and form of Sat-Chita-Ananda.

When Arjuna was confused and deluded, he humbly surrendered himself to Krishna as a disciple and sought Krishna's guidance. Deep in his heart, Arjuna took refuge in Krishna as the Supreme Sadguru.

Here Lord Krishna accepted Arjuna as his disciple and played his divine role like a good friend, charioteer and Sadguru by showing Arjuna the path of Dharma.

Krishna spoke to Arjuna in the form of the Supreme Divine Consciousness, as the Lord of the entire Universe and as a creator, protector and destroyer all at the same time. Krishna mentions that he dwells in all beings and all souls.

How was Bhagavad Gita Recorded or Written and bought forward to us?

Maharishi Vyasa iss one of the key characters, a mystic Sadhu or Rishi possessing many mystic and yogic powers. According to the Bhagavat Purana, Vyasa was also an incarnation of Vishnu.

He was the one who fathered Dhritarashtra, Pandu and Vidur, which he did due to very compelling reasons for the sake of the continuation of progeny in the Kuru Kingdom, upon his mother's request. Thus he was the grandfather of both the Kauravas (Sons of Dhritarashtra) and the Pandavas (sons of Pandu).

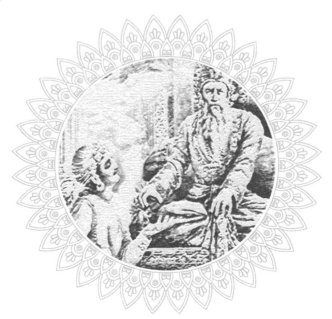

He was a great personality and a knower of Trikala (past, present and future). He would present himself physically at most critical places and times amidst his kin, in order to give them solace when in trouble and guide them on dharma.

He was a witness and also a historian of the entire Mahabharata story.

Since King Dhritarashtra was blind, he could not participate in the War.I In order to keep him informed of the day-to-day developments and happenings in the war, Vyasa gave special powers of visualisation ('doordarshan') to Sanjaya, a personal assistant/ minister of King Dhritarashtra to remotely witness all that was happening in the Kurukshetra war in order to narrate them. The power also included reading the thoughts of the people who were engaged in the war.

Sanjaya, using the divine powers blessed to him by Vyasa, narrated every minute detail of the happenings at the war front (as a flashback) to the blind king.

The Bhagavad Gita portion of the Mahabharata in fact starts with Dhritarashtra asking Sanjaya to tell him what his own sons and the Pandavas, assembled at the battlefield, were doing. Sanjaya begins his narration of the scenario where both sides were ready to begin the war. It was then that Arjuna asked Krishna to take his chariot to the middle where he could see his opponents standing ready and geared up to fight them. Subsequent happenings and the dialog between Krishna and Arjuna (which formed the Bhagavad Gita) was narrated to Dhritarashtra by Sanjaya. Sanjaya continued with the narration of every detail and happening in the war subsequently.

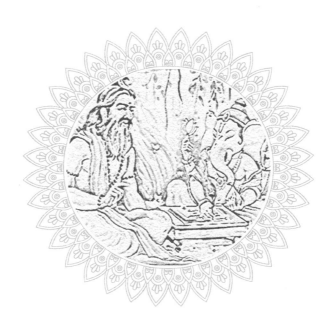

Vyasa dictating the Mahabharata for Lord Ganesha to write it.

Much later in life, after the period of the Pandavas and Kauravas, Sage Vyasa formed in his mind the entire story of Mahabharata as a grand Itihasa which was too monumental a work for him to put into writing. Conceding to his prayers, Lord Brahma engaged Lord Ganesha to write this grand epic on palm leaves based on the dictation of Vyasa.

The present version of the Mahabharata, as available to us, contains some 24000 verses. The Bhagavad Gita is placed in the middle of the Mahabharata as part of Book 6 - Bhishma Parva - spreading across 18 chapters (Chapters 25 to 42). The Gita contains 700 slokas (verses).

Vyasa's Mahabharata text, that we have today, is not actually a direct narration of Vyasa but it is understood to be narrated by Ugrasrava, who was the son of Romaharshana Rishi, surnamed Souti to the rishis of Naimisharanya!

The Vyasa Bharata story was heard by him from Maharishi Vaisampayana (a disciple of Vyasa) as he narrated it to King Janamejaya (Grandson of Abhimanyu and great-grandson of Arjuna) during a Sarpa Yagna in the august presence of Sage Vyasa himself.

Thus, the Bhagavad Gita (and Mahabharata) as the authentic Sanskrit script available in the present form is from Souti (Ugrasrava) as heard by him from Rishi Vaisampayana. Thus this specific text's period of origin is at least about 60 to 100 years after the actual Kurukshetra war.

How Krishna managed to counsel Arjuna

Krishna managed to counsel and convince Arjuna by teaching him lessons on Karma Yoga (doing all his actions without the desire for the fruit – niskama karma). Further Krishna reminds Arjuna of his Dharma as a Kshatriya (warrior with the ability to protect others) to fight against the negative forces.

Krishna explains the eternity of our atman or soul (jivatma) and higher truths are really about the Atman (self) and Parmatman (divine self).

He explained the idea of selfless action, surrendering fruits to the Divine, which would make him free from any guilt from the wrong perception of killing people in a war.

Further Krishna explains Jnana Yoga, Samkhya Yoga, Dhyana Yoga, Raja Yoga, Bhakti Yoga to help Arjuna understand various paths leading us to self-realisation. Krishna holds Karma Yoga as the highest path as we can never be free of creating or doing Karma.

Krishna explained the various deep spiritual wisdom (adhyatma vijnana) from the Upanishads and other scriptures in a simple way that Arjuna could understand.

He revealed to Arjuna about His divinity. He revealed his Vishvarupa (cosmic divine form) to Arjuna, clearing him of all doubts. Arjuna realised Krishna's all-encompassing power, and he surrendered himself to Krishna completely and acted as per his instructions.

He got back his lost confidence and stood up valiantly to fight the war to its logical finish.

What makes the Bhagavad Gita and Mahabharat authentic?

It sounds like such a tough job to preserve the original manuscript of these ancient texts like Bhagavad Gita, written around 5000BC. Many of these teachings are preserved traditionally in Guru-Shisya-Paramaparai as well as in 'Pothis' (ancient poetic texts) written on palm leaves all over India - with some 'Patha Bhedas' (slight variations in texts).

It was the Bhandarkar Oriental Research Institute, Pune, that took on the monumental project of compiling a Critical Edition of the Mahabharata. This edition was prepared through the painstaking efforts of scholars like V. S. Sukhtankar, S. K. Belvalkar, S. K. De, Prof. Dr. R. N. Dandekar over five decades consulting 1,259 manuscripts. The task took 50 years, starting from 1917.

Taking into consideration these available manuscripts, Prof. Shripad Krishna Belvalkar published an 'Authentic Version' (critical edition) of the Bhagavad-Gita in November, 1941.

It is also worth noting the work done by Gitapress Gorakhapur, with a large team of scholars and Sanskrita masters, to publish their editions of the Mahabharata and Bhagavat Gita, preserving its authenticity.

What Makes the Bhagavad Gita so Important among Yoga and Hindu followers?

The teachings of the Bhagavad Gita taught to Arjuna by Lord Krishna were not only meant for Arjuna. Lord Krishna took this opportunity to bless mankind with these spiritual teachings to help foster peace, love, compassion, harmony and righteousness along with self-realisation or Kaivalya.

These teachings can be seen as scientifically organised mental, emotional and spiritual counselling. There is an answer to all our inner battles, conflicts, confusions and delusions. The Bhagavad Gita explains the essence of the Vedic lifestyle in concepts of Karma and Dharma (righteousness) and attaining Moksha or Liberation. It emphasises the importance of fulfilling the purpose of life and facing all the ups and downs of life without being a victim, to live our life in balance and equanimity (Samatva).

The Vedas and Upanishads offer Karma Yoga and Jnana Yoga as two separate paths. Karma Yoga is doing our duties without seeking fruits and offering it all to the divine purpose. Jnana Yoga is the path of wisdom, knowing the ultimate reality of Atma and Parmatman as one, and everything else that is subject to change as Maya or Illusion. The Bhagavad Gita brings these two paths together and explains how one without the other is not fruitful. Also, Krishna gave all the teachings to Arjuna in a much simpler language, easily understood by everyone.

The Bhagavad Gita is available to each and every individual that is interested in the greatest spiritual wisdom of Sanatan Dharma, regardless of their cast, colour and religion.

18 Chapters of the Bhagavad Gita

Chapter 1:   Arjuna's Grief or Despair; Arjuna Vishada Yoga

Chapter 2:   Arjuna's Enquiry, Samkhya Yoga

Chapter 3:   Karma Yoga, Yoga of Action

Chapter 4:   Renunciation of Action; Jnana Karma Sanyasa Yoga

Chapter 5:   Yoga of True Renunciation; Karma Sanyasa Yoga

Chapter 6:   Yoga of Meditation; Dhyana Yoga

Chapter 7:   Knowledge and Wisdom; Jnana Vijnana Yoga

Chapter 8:   Eternal Brahman; Akshara Brahma Yoga

Chapter 9:   The Royal Secret; Raja-vidya or Raja Yoga

Chapter 10: Divine Glories of Bhagavan; Vibhuti Yoga

Chapter 11: The Vision of Cosmic Form; Vishwarupa Darshana Yoga

Chapter 12: Yoga of Devotion; Bhakti Yoga

Chapter 13: The Field and Its Knower; Kshetra Kshetrajna Vibhagha Yoga

Chapter 14: The Yoga of Gunas; Gunatraya Vibhaga Yoga

Chapter 15: Yoga of the Supreme Spirit; Purushottama Yoga

Chapter 16: Divine and Devilish Estates; Daiva Asura Sampat Vibhaga Yoga

Chapter 17: The Threefold Path; Shraddhatraya Vibhaga Yoga

Chapter 18: Liberation Through Renunciation; Moksha Sanyasa Yoga

Chapter 1: Arjuna's Grief or Despair; Arjuna Vishada Yoga

The Bhagavad Gita teachings begin at the very beginning of the Kurkshetra War, where Arjuna found himself in grief, despair, confusion and delusion. He was unable to see what is right for him to do as to take part in the war would involve killing his own family members, friends and relatives. Here Arjuna represents all seeking minds looking for answers for our life problems.

Chapter 2: Arjuna's Enquiry, Samkhya Yoga

The teachings of the Bhagavad Gita begin in chapter 2 with Krishna guiding us through Samkhya Yoga where he explains the immortality and eternity of the Atman or soul and changing nature of the body. Krishna explains that the Atman is not subject to any change, birth, death or any suffering.

Verse 48: Remaining steadfast in yoga, oh! Dhanañjaya, perform actions, abandoning attachment, remaining the same to success and failure alike. This evenness of mind is known as yoga.

Chapter 3: Karma Yoga, Yoga of Action

In this Arjuna recognises that he wants to attain Moksha, Liberation, enlightenment, and nothing less and asks Krishna why he should take part in war instead of taking the path of Sanyasa or renunciation.

In the third chapter Krishna explains the nature of Karma and asks Arjuna to fulfil his Dharma and take part in the war without desiring the fruits (niskam karma). Here Krishna explains the nature of desires and likes and dislikes.

Verse 5: Indeed no one ever exists for even a second without performing action because everyone, being helpless, is made to perform action by the gunas (tamas, rajas and sattva) born of prakriti.

Chapter 4: Renunciation of Action; Jnana Karma Sanyasa Yoga

In this chapter Krishna begins with detailing the roots of Sanatan Dharma and Yogic Teachings and details the idea or Avataras or incarnations. An incarnation is Parmatman or Supreme Self in human body, like Krishna himself to establish humanity and Dharma or righteousness in society.

Further Krishna explains how Atman or oneself can be totally free of all the actions and remain unbounded of karma, time and space. Krishna also explains reality at various levels like empirical reality (the sun, moon, stars, birds, trees etc), the subjective reality (individual perception and experiences), Ultimate reality or Brahman.

Verse 24: The means of offering is Brahman. The oblation is Brahman, offered by Brahman, into the fire, which is Brahman. Brahman is indeed to be reached by him who sees everything as Brahman.

Chapter 5: Yoga of True Renunciation; Karma Sanyasa Yoga

Arjuna still believes that renunciation is the key to Moksha or liberation. So far Krishna has praised both Karma Yoga and

Sanyasa Yoga, so in this chapter Arjuna asks "which path is better?" Both lead to liberation but these paths present two very different life paths.

Krishna explains that Sanyasa, although it may look like an easier, faster path, is actually much more difficult, as there is a certain depth of understanding needed before one can truly be a sanyasi. Karma yoga actually prepares one for sanyasa. The Karma Yoga path is living our whole life, moment by moment and 'doing our best and leaving the rest -karmeshu kaushalam'.

Verse 11: Giving up attachment, karma-yogis perform action purely (without attachment) with the body, mind, intellect, and also by the senses, for the purification of the mind.

Chapter 6: Yoga of Meditation; Dhyana Yoga

In this chapter Krishna teaches us how to focus our mind and also details the nature of the mind. Here Krishna advises us to become the witnessing awareness and remain mindful to each and every moment to transform our old habitual patterns known as Samaskaras.

Krishna describes sitting meditation, in a quiet, clean and uncluttered place, to purify the mind. He again uses the terms sthira and sthitah, to indicate a sense of undisturbed steadiness.

Verses 34 and 35: Arjuna says, "As we all know, Krishna, the mind is 'agitation', a strong, well rooted tyrant. I think of it as impossible to control as the wind." Krishna replies, "No doubt, O mighty-armed (Arjuna), the agitated mind is very difficult to control. But, oh son of Kunti, by abhyaasa (practice) and vairagyam (objectivity), it is mastered.

Chapter 7: Knowledge and Wisdom; Jnana Vijnana Yoga

Here Jnana signifies an indirect knowledge from various sources while Vijnana applies for individual experience of Atman and Parmatman as ultimate reality.

Krishna tells Arjuna that this knowledge is rare in the world. Very few seek it at this level, and of the ones who do, still fewer come to full realisation.

Krishna introduces the term Prakrti and explains the manifest universe as apara prakrti, the world of form, the elements etc. Para prakrti is the unchanging source or primordial cause of the apara prakrti.

Krishna explains the law of creation, sustenance and dissolution. He mentions that, "I am the cause of the entire creation and its ultimate dissolution."

Verse 1: Krishna Said: O Paartha, please listen to the way in which you will know me totally, without any doubt, by living yoga, with a mind committed to Me and having surrendered to Me.

Chapter 8: Eternal Brahman; Akshara Brahma Yoga

Arjuna begins chapter 8 by asking about Brahman and what happens at the time of death. Krishna explains to Arjuna that contemplation on Parameshvara and also the chanting of OM are ways to realise Brahman.

Krishna explains the nature the celestial realms (Lokas) and cosmic time scales (Yugas), and the cycles of birth and death to help Arjuna distinguish between the world of maya, or change, and the eternal or unchanging Brahman. Brahma-vidyaa, Ultimate knowledge of Brahman, alone brings liberation.

Verse 8: O! Partha, reflecting as he was taught, with a mind endowed with the practice of yoga, with a mind that does not stray to anything else, he reaches the limitless, self-effulgent SELF (Purusha).

Chapter 9: The Royal Secret; Raja-vidya or Raja Yoga

The knowledge is said to be secret because even if you hear the teachings, it is rarely understood unless we are ready for them. Also, this true wisdom or Vijnana is not subject to our sensory experience like the worldly or material wisdom. We can attain it with total commitment, compassion, faith, grace and devotion. A mature mind is needed for spiritual knowledge and these virtues, when cultivated, lead to maturity.

Verse 14: Those who are always focussed on Me, and making their best efforts, whose commitment is firm and who remain surrendered to Me with devotion, who are always united to ME (with a loving heart), I am always with them.

Chapter 10: Divine Glories of Bhagavan; Vibhuti Yoga

The Bhagavan, the Divinity is everything and all-pervading. Lord Krishna is referred to as Bhagavan throughout the Gita. Bhagavan means 'one who has bhaga, the six aspects of wholesomeness, or the six absolute virtues'. These are all riches, all strength, all fame, all beauty, all knowledge, and all renunciation. Bhagavan is not only all forms, all manifestations, all creation, but also the source, the creator, who remains unchanged, aham sthitah, all along the transforming universe.

Verse 19: Well now, O! Best of the Kurus, Arjuna. I will tell you My divine glories in keeping with their importance; because there is no end to a detailed description of My glories.

Chapter 11: The Vision of Cosmic Form; Vishwarupa Darshana Yoga

In this Chapter Lord Krishna blesses Arjuna with the divine vision (Divya Darshan) of his Cosmic Form or Vishwarupa. Here it is explained that we cannot experience divinity with our senses and mundane mind.

Verse 55: Among all people, the one who does all action for My sake, for whom I am paramount, who is devoted to Me, free from attachment and free from enmity, he comes to Me, Arjuna.

Chapter 12: Yoga of Devotion; Bhakti Yoga

In this chapter Krishna details the path of Bhakti Yoga. Offering all our actions to Ishwara, or the divine, and service to humanity or dharma is known as Bhakti.

Krishna explains that it is the attitude with which one performs the daily activities that leads to self-knowledge. This attitude is devotion or bhakti.

Verses 8 and 9: In Me alone you may place the mind; into Me you will make the intellect enter. Thereafter there is no doubt that you will abide in Me alone. Then (if) you are not able to absorb your mind steadily in Me, then through the practice of yoga may you reach Me Arjuna.

Chapter 13: The Field and Its Knower; Kshetra Kshetrajna Vibhagha Yoga

In this chapter Krishna details the nature of purusha and prakriti, the knower and the known. Krishnaa begins by discussing Kshetra and Kshetrajña because those words do not have the connotations imposed upon purusha and prakriti by the Sankhyas. Krishna also discusses jnana, especially in relation to the values and attitudes of a mind that is mature and ready for knowledge (brahma-vidya).

Verse 12: What is to be known, that I will tell clearly, knowing, which one gains immortality, that Brahman, which, it is known, has no beginning, is limitless, neither existent (as an object) nor non-existent.

Chapter 14: The Yoga of Gunas; Gunatraya Vibhaga Yoga

Krishna in this chapter describes the process of creation, the known universe, the birth of Prakrti and the Tri-Gunas. These three Gunas are Sattva, Rajas and Tamas. Here Krishna teaches us how to transcend these Gunas to attain liberation.

Verse 9: O! Bhaarata, sattva binds in the form of absolute bliss, rajas in the form of action and material attainments. But tamas, covering knowledge, binds indeed in the form of inertia and sensual indulgence.

Chapter 15: Yoga of the Supreme Spirit; Purushottama Yoga

This a short chapter, including 20 slokas detailing the tree of Samsara, the nature of the Jiva, (the individual being), the subtle body and reincarnation. It further explains how to develop our mind to maturity, to experience the all-illuminating light, the perishable and the imperishable.

Verse 15: And I have entered the hearts of all. From Me (have come) memory, knowledge, and forgetfulness. I am alone the one to be known by all the Vedas and I alone am the author of the Vedanta and the know-er of the Vedas.

Chapter 16: Divine and Devilish Estates; Daiva Asura Sampat Vibhaga Yoga

In chapter sixteen Lord Krishna uses Devas and Asuras to highlight qualities to aspire to and qualities to avoid. Spiritual wealth, the wealth of the devas, accumulates as one nurtures certain values and these values need to be understood, not just mindlessly followed.

Verse 22: A man who is free from these three gates to darkness, Arjuna, follows what is good for himself. Because of that he reaches the highest goal.

Chapter 17: The Threefold Path of Sraddha; Shraddhatraya Vibhaga Yoga

In this Chapter Krishna explains the Path of three Shraddhas – faith that we follow or temperament or attitude towards life values we live with. These are tamasic, rajasic and sattvic. This explains the types of food we eat, activities we take part in, and life choices we make. Krishna explains the moral and ethical virtues of Yamas and Niyamas and om tat sat, the ultimate expression of Brahman.

Verse 16: Mental cheerfulness, cheerfulness in expression, inner silence, mastery over the mind, clean intent – this (these together) is called mental discipline.

Chapter 18: Liberation Through Renunciation; Moksha Sanyasa Yoga

This is the longest chapter, 78 verses and Krishna's teaching ends with a restatement of the previous teachings. "Giving up all karmas, take refuge in Me alone. I will free you from all karma; do not grieve".

In this chapter Krishna returns back to fundamental teachings of Karma, Sanyasa and Moksha and details the Sanyasa Marga or path of renunciation.

Reference and Resources:
1. Bhagavad Gita by Gitapress Gorakhapur, India.
2. Yoga Step by Step by Swamiji Dr Gitananda Giriji.
3. Bhagavad Gita as It is by Swami Prabhupad.
4. The Bhagavad Gita by Ekanath Easwaran.
5. The Teachings of Bhagavad Gita by Swami Dayananda Saraswati
6. https://en.wikipedia.org/wiki/Bhagavad_Gita
7. https://www.bhagavad-gita.org/
8. https://www.holy-bhagavad-gita.org/

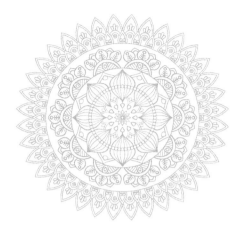

Chapter 1
Arjuna's Grief or Despair; Arjuna Vishada Yoga

The greatest war of Mahabharata was fought between the Pandavas (five brothers representing righteousness and all their supporters) and the Kauravas (representing the 100 sons of King Dhratrashtra and their supporters in injustice and immoral acts).

At the very beginning of this war, the greatest warrior and archer Arjuna surrenders to Lord Krishna. Krishna is the Divine incarnation of Vishnu, and Arjuna sees him as his friend, charioteer, guide, guru and the divine.

In chapter one Arjuna explains his problems, pain, confusion and lack of ability to make the decision if he should take part in the battle or not. He was unsure of what was right and what was wrong for him. He requests Krishna to guide his soul and show him the right path whether to fight or renounce and live like an ascetic or sage. The teachings of the Bhagavad Gita, these most scientific and practical teachings for all humankind to live and grow spiritually by, were instructed to Arjuna.

Chapter one in many ways is most important as "One needs to realise and/or accept the problem, before one can find a solution." As in the medical profession, to prescribe a medicine, first a doctor needs to follow the diagnosis process. One needs to clearly know the problem in order to offer a solution. In Yogic Sadhana or our evolutionary journey, self-enquiry or questions are in many ways far more important than the answers. Our divine Guru or teacher can only teach us what we are willing to learn or follow.

Arjuna is not only suffering with the problems or confusion and despair, but he also accepts them and is asking Lord Krishna to guide him or show him the light. The Gita provides practical solutions to all our Samasarik (worldly) problems at a physical, mental, social, and spiritual level.

Once one realises the problem or pain in life, he or she must also possess sincere desire or longing (tivra-mumuksha; tivra - sincere and mumuksha - desire or longing) to be free of suffering. This can lead one to dedicated and fruitful sadhana (practice) and yoga (union or oneness of body, mind, senses and soul).

Further one also needs to accept his or her limited knowledge or understanding, let go of the ego of intelligence and seek for guidance or help. This is exactly what Arjuna does at the beginning of the battle in Chapter 1. He surrenders himself to Krishna, explaining his state of confusion, illusion and lack of clarity in knowing what is right and what is wrong. He surrenders himself as a Shisya (sincere student) and prepares the ideal state for his Guru (teacher or guide who leads one from darkness to light) Krishna. This is how the higher teachings of the Gita manifest.

In the whole first chapter and the first part of the second chapter, Arjuna explains all the problems. The problems of Samsara here are as follows:

Raga - Attachment, desire to seek for pleasure
Soka or Visada - Grief, despair
Moha - delusion, or attraction for material things.

When we are not happy with ourselves, we seek external aids for happiness. This leads to dependence, attachment. Now as we know, all these possessions are impermanent, this causes fear. Also, if we don't get what we desire, we feel unhappy, angry or emotional. We lose peace and balance of mind. When our mind is at trouble or disturbed, we make poor choices and decisions. This complicates the situation further. This is just the simplest example of all the problems of this Samasara.

In the first 20 verses of Chapter one there is a description of both the armies and the great warriors arrayed for the battle. Then all the commanders of the Kauravas, Bhisma and others, Lord Krishna, Arjuna and others blow their conches, signaling for the commencement of the battle.

At this point Arjuna requests Krishna, his charioteer, to take his chariot into the middle of the two armies, so he can see them all before the battle begins. Lord Krishna brings the chariot into the middle and asks Arjuna to survey the army. (BG 1.21-25)

Up to this point Prince Arjuna was convinced that his cousins were unrighteous, and it was his duty to battle against them to establish righteousness as a Kshatriya (cast of warriors, who fight to protect others).

At this moment he lost his mental ability to be discerning (viveka) and found himself trapped in attachment of relationships. Instead of seeing his Dharma, he sees his beloved kith and kin in opposition. This attachment results into grief, and delusion. (BG 1.26-30)

In the next five verses Arjuna explains his intense grief and says why he would participate in such a battle, killing all these people who are related to him, some of whom have loved and blessed him with their knowledge, wisdom, and skills on life like Bhishma, his Guru Dronachariya etc. He explains now that he desires for nothing, so why should he fight? He further queries what pleasure it will bring even if he were to acquire all three worlds after killing all these people.

He further mentions that even though the Kauravas are overpowered by their greed and selfishness and have lost their Viveka, why should we who still are able to use our reasoning (viveka) and know what is right, knowing that killing and battle is not good for anyone, fight. (BG 1.31-36)

In the next few verses Arjuna uses some scriptural references to support his views and delusion. He further mentions to Krishna that if families are destroyed, Dharma or righteous attitude to fulfil duties will perish. This will further destroy the moral and ethical values of women and children left behind unprotected as the result of battle. He says it is better for him to be killed by his enemies when he is unarmed. He surrenders at the feet of Lord Krishna for guidance and puts his bow down sorrowfully.

In Summary this chapter deals with:
1. Descriptions and preparations of both armies (verses 1 to 20)
2. Arjuna's confused mind due to raga (attachment), and Soka (grief) (verses 21 to 34)
3. Arjuna's delusion (verses 35 to 47)

This chapter is known as Arjuna-Visada-Yoga as this whole chapter deals with Arjuna's grief.

Arjuna's Grief or Despair; Arjuna Vishada Yoga

BG 1.1: Dhritarashtra said: O Sanjay, after gathering on the holy battlefield of Kurukshetra, with their desire to fight, what are my sons and the sons of Pandu doing?

BG 1.2: Sanjay said: On observing the Pandava army ready for battle, King Duryodhan approached his teacher Dronacharya, and said the following words.

BG 1.3: Duryodhan said: Respected master! Observe the mighty army of the sons of Pandu, so expertly arranged for battle by your own blessed disciple, the son of King Drupad.

BG 1.4-6: Witness how in their orders are many powerful warriors, like Yuyudhan, Virat, and Drupad, exercising mighty bows and equal in military prowess to Bheem and Arjun. There are also accomplished heroes like Dhrishtaketu, Chekitan, the gallant King of Kashi, Purujit, Kuntibhoj, and Shaibya— all the best of warriors. In their defences, they also have the courageous Yudhamanyu, the gallant Uttamauja, the son of Subhadra, and the sons of Draupadi, who are all great warriors.

BG 1.7: O greatest of Brahmins, hear too about the chief warriors on our side, who are especially competent to lead. I now narrate to you about those warriors on our side.

BG 1.8: There are great people like yourself, Bheeshma, Karna, Kripa, Ashwatthama, Vikarn, and Bhurishrava, who are ever victorious in battle.

BG 1.9: Also, there are many other heroic warriors, who are prepared to sacrifice their lives for my sake. They are all skilled in the art of warfare and equipped with various kinds of weapons and war skills.

BG 1.10: The strength of our army is boundless, and we are safely marshalled by Grandsire Bheeshma, while the strength of the Pandava army, carefully marshalled by Bheem, is inadequate.

BG 1.11: Therefore, I call upon all the generals of the Kaurava army now to fully support Grandsire Bheeshma, even as you defend your respective strategic points.

BG 1.12: Then, the grandsire, the oldest man of the Kuru dynasty, the glorious patriarch Bheeshma, roared like a lion, and blew his conch shell loudly, to bring joy to Duryodhan.

BG 1.13: Thereafter, conches, kettledrums, bugles, trumpets, and horns suddenly blared forth, and their combined sound was overwhelming and frightening for weak hearts.

BG 1.14: Then, from among the Pandava army, Madhava or Krishna and Arjuna blew their divine conch shells from their glorious chariot drawn by white horses.

BG 1.15: Hrishikesh (Krishna) blew his conch shell known as Panchajanya, and Arjun blew the Devadutta. Bheem, the voracious eater and performer of extraordinary tasks, blew his mighty conch known as Paundra.

BG 1.16-18: King Yudhishthir blew the conch Anantavijay, while Nakul and Sahadev blew the Sughosh and Manipushpak. The excellent archer and king of Kashi, the great warrior Shikhandi, Dhrishtadyumna, Virat, and the invincible Satyaki, Drupad, the five sons of Draupadi, and the mighty-armed Abhimanyu, son of Subhadra, all blew their respective conch shells, O Ruler of the earth.

BG 1.19: The tremendous sounds of conches and other instruments resounded across the sky and the earth, and traumatised the hearts of your sons, O Dhritarasthra.

BG 1.20: At this point, Arjuna, the son of Pandu, who had the insignia of Hanuman on the flag of his chariot, took up his bow. Seeing your sons arrayed against him, O King, Arjun then spoke the following words to Shree Krishna.

BG 1.21-22: Arjun said: O Trustworthy One, please take my chariot into the middle of both armies, so that I may look at the warriors grouped for battle, whom I must fight in this great battle.

BG 1.23: I desire to see those who have come here to support the evil-minded son of Dhritarasthra, wishing to please him.

BG 1.24: Sanjay said: O Dhritarasthra, having thus been addressed by Arjun, the conqueror of sleep, Shree Krishna then drew the magnificent chariot into the middle of the two armies.

BG 1.25: In the presence of Bheeshma, Dronacharya, and all the other kings, Shree Krishna said: O Parth, observe these Kuru warriors assembled here.

BG 1.26: There, Arjun could see stationed in both armies, his uncles, grandfathers, teachers, maternal uncles, brothers, cousins, sons, nephews, grand-nephews, friends, fathers-in-law, and well-wishers.

BG 1.27: Seeing all his family members and relatives against him at the battlefield, Arjun, the son of Kunti, was overwhelmed with compassion, and with deep sorrow, spoke the following words.

BG 1.28: Arjun said: O Krishna, seeing my own kinsmen grouped for battle here and intent on killing each other, my limbs are trembling, and my mouth is drying up.

BG 1.29-31: My whole-body trembles; my hair is standing on end. My bow, the Gandiv, is slipping away from my hand, and my skin is burning in sorrow. My mind is in dilemma and revolving in confusion; I am unable to hold myself steady any longer. O Krishna, killer of the Keshi demon, I only see omens of misfortune. I do not foresee how any good can come from killing my own beloved ones in this battle.

BG 1.32-33: O Krishna, I do not desire the victory, or joy in acquiring the kingdom. Of what benefit will be a kingdom, pleasures, or even life itself, when the very persons for whom we desire, are standing before us for battle?

BG 1.34-35: Teachers, fathers, sons, grandfathers, maternal uncles, grandsons, fathers-in-law, grand-nephews, brothers-in-law, and other family members are present here, staking their lives and riches. O Madhusudan, I do not wish to kill them, even if they kill me. What satisfaction will we attain from acquiring over the three worlds, after killing the sons of Dhristarashtra, what to speak of this Earth?

BG 1.36-37: O Divine Sustaining power of all living beings, what pleasure will we attain from killing the sons of Dhritarasthra? Even though they may be invaders, sin will certainly come upon us if we kill them. Hence, it does not suit us to kill our own cousins, the sons of Dhritarashtra, and friends. O Madhav (Krishna), how can we hope to be happy by killing our own kinsmen?

BG 1.38-39: Their minds are caught by greed and they see no wrong in destroying their relatives or inflicting treachery upon friends. Yet, O Janardan (Krishna), why should we not turn away from this sin, as we can clearly see the crime in killing our relatives?

BG 1.40: When an empire is destroyed, its civilisations and traditions get vanquished, and the rest of the family members become involved in adharma or unrighteous acts.

BG 1.41: With the predominance of corruption, O Krishna, the women of the family become immoral; and from the immorality of women, O descendent of Vrishni, unwanted offspring are born.

BG 1.42: An increase in unwanted children results in hell on earth for the lives of those from both sides in a battle. Deprived of the sacrificial offerings, the descendants of such corrupt families also fall.

BG 1.43: Through the evil deeds of those who destroy the family tradition and thus give rise to unwanted offspring, a variety of social, family and cultural welfare activities are ruined.

BG 1.44: O Janardan (Krishna), I have learned from the masters that those who destroy family traditions dwell in hell for an indefinite period of time.

BG 1.45-46: Alas! How strange it is that our minds are set to perform this great sin. Driven by the desire for royal pleasures, we are determined to kill our own people. It will be better if the sons of Dhritarashtra kill me while I am unarmed and unresisting on the battlefield with their weapons.

BG 1.47: Sanjay said: Speaking this, Arjun places his bow and arrow sideways, and lapses into the seat of his chariot, with his mind in distress and overwhelmed with grief.

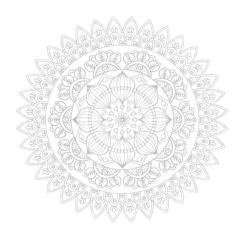

Chapter 2
Arjuna's Enquiry, Samkhya Yoga

The first chapter in the Bhagavad Gita details Arjuna's grief (soka) caused by attachment (raga) and delusion (moha). After analysing his problems and pain, he concluded that withdrawing from the war was the solution.

In the beginning of the second chapter Arjuna explains his situation further and uses some wise references, trying to convince Lord Krishna that his decision to not follow his duty of taking part in war to protect righteousness is correct. This shows Arjuna's weakness of attachment as a problem which cannot be solved by superficial knowledge and awareness. This leads Arjuna to take refuge under the guidance of Krishna as his Guru in order to seek answers. (BG 2.1-9) This is actually one of the key issues in the Yoga World in our modern age. Everyone wants to start their yogic journey from meditation and samadhi itself.

Arjuna becomes a shisya (student or disciple) by his genuine refuge and seeking heart to find solutions from Lord Krishna, and Krishna becomes his divine Guru or Teacher. In Yogic, Hindu and Vedic traditions, divine or spiritual teachings can only take place once a profound, loving, respectful, faithful, and service-based relationship is established between Guru-Shishya, or Guru-Chela (student-teacher). The teachings of Lord Krishna in the Bhagavad Gita are scientific tools of remedy for all our mental, emotional, social and spiritual problems, and they begin from verse 10 of chapter 2.

It is also known in Vedic teachings that "when a man or woman awakens the seeker in himself or herself, the Guru or Teacher manifests in his or her life at that moment."

The first teaching of Krishna for Arjuna in Verse 11 of chapter 2 was, "Oh, Arjuna because of delusion caused by ignorance, you are wrongly thinking that you can kill all these people or anyone of them can kill you. The true nature of Atman (soul) is immortal. From its Adhyatmink-dristi, true nature of existence, the soul is not subject to any changes. Only the body goes through all the changes. The soul is not the doer (Karta) nor the enjoyer or consumer (bhokta). Krishna says, for that reason, why should you refuse to fight." (BG 2.12-25)

Krishna further mentions that even if the Atman is impermanent, even then Arjuna should not deviate from his Dharma (duty) to fight. What manifests or appears will have to disappear or dispose back to its source to complete the cycle. Krishna asks Arjuna to accept the reality of change. In reality, change is the most beautiful aspect of creation and evolution. Krishna further mentions that one who is born, must die. The body grows from birth into youth, from youth to adult, from adult to old age and then it perishes, but the soul remains eternal all through this process. So, if death is inevitable, why should Arjuna grieve over it. (BG 2.26-30)

Further Krishna explains to Arjuna from his dharmika-dristi (duty point of view), his duty as a Kshatriya. Arjuna as a warrior should fight if it is necessary to establish law and order. He also mentions that this fight is necessary to kill all these people from a social point of view (samajik-dristi), in order to bring about peace and justice. Krishna says: "oh Bharata, you should not hesitate for a righteous cause". Krishna says to Arjuna that he will not only lose his path to self-realisation by not taking part in this war, but he will also incur sin, and for that reason he must follow his duty to fight. (BG 2.31-32)

Further Krishna explains it to Arjuna from his worldly point of view (laukika dristi). Krishna says that he is a great warrior, a prince and a great role model for many others. In that case if he should withdraw from the war people will see him as a coward. Also, many people will take his action as an example to follow. Krishna says then that he must fight to establish a good example of following the duty for generations to come as well as to protect his own reputation. With these examples, Krishna encourages Arjuna to take part in the fight. (BG 2. 33-38) and concludes the first part of his divine teaching. Krishna calls this sankhya-yoga (39).

Some important Samkhya Yoga teachings of chapter 2

Atman or soul is eternal (atma-nityam), like our body changes from child to youth, adult to old, our souls also change –

changing body just like we change our old clothes. A firm Sadhaka should not fear or grieve over this change. (BG. 2.13) The only way to attain freedom from all the suffering is by remaining firm in equanimity regarding both painful and pleasurable situations (Samatvam). (BG 2.15)

All that is subject to change is unreal, and what is real is always eternal. All the material objects and subjects of sensory experiences are unreal, so why suffer for what is known by yogis as ever changing? (BG 2.16)

The Atman or soul is eternal and not subject to any changes. Fire cannot burn it, water cannot wet it, air cannot blow it, heat cannot dry it, and sword cannot cut it. The Atman or soul is unborn and hence never dies. Just like we change the old clothes, the soul changes body. (BG 2.20-23)

This is one of the most elaborate definitions of soul, atman or consciousness. We can translate this into modern words as the "domain of non-local, acausal, timeless, quantum conscious-intellectual-living force".

Further in this chapter Krishna teaches Arjuna about Yoga, which brings the wisdom of Samkhya Yoga into practice. Krishna says for one who knows Samkhya and practices it even a little, Yoga will protect that Sadhaka. If we follow our dharma or fulfil our duties, our dharma will protect us. One should remain single-pointed, otherwise our mind, will and thoughts will be multi-branched. (BG 2.40-42)

In the next few verses Krishna explains that doing our duties is more important than following religious rituals seeking for heavenly pleasures and/or material desires. These people can never attain Samadhi or Liberation. (BG 2.43-44)

Krishna explains that all our actions, thoughts, feelings and emotions are driven from the tri-gunas (three primary qualities) - sattva (purity, light), rajas (action, passion) and tamas (inertia, darkness). To remain in Sattva or pure state of bliss, one needs to be free from the effects of opposites - of liking-disliking, pain-pleasure, hot-cold.

Do your Karma or fulfil your duties Arjuna, without desiring for their fruits (niskam karma). Stay focused and follow your dharma without attachment and maintaining balance in success and failure. Any action done for the sake of fruit is the cause of Karmic attachment. (BG 2.47-49)

Using the Viveka (wisdom of reasoning and righteousness), one who remains mindful (Jagruka), maintains equanimity (samtvam) and practices the yoga of skill in action (yogah-karmeshu-kausalam), he or she becomes free from all the good and bad actions and their fruits (karma-phala mukti). Once a wise person abandons all his desires towards the fruits of his actions (niskam Karma), he or she attains freedom from the cycles of birth-life-and death. (BG 2.50-51)

Krishna says that a calm and tranquil mind will soon withdraw from worldly attractions, turning instead towards the Atman. When one establishes his mind or awareness in the peaceful or joyful Atman, he attains liberation or self-realisation. (BG 2.52-53)

Here Arjuna asks Krishna, please tell me the characteristics of the great yogi or master (sthiti-prajna) who is firmly established in Self-Knowledge (atma-jnana). (BG 2.53)

Knowledge and intellect are only fruitful when one can bring them into practice, also stabilisinges and assimilating his or her mind. Krishna here mentions two important practices - control or discipline of mind and the sense organs, and contemplation on these universal divine teachings. Through this knowledge becomes our experience. (BG 2.58-61). If we don't follow these teachings our mind and sense organs will become enslaved to the concerns of the sense organs and desires, and this will lead the Sadhaka away from the spiritual path of evolution. (BG 2.62-62)

Lord Krishna further explains the character of Sthita-Prajna (one who has mastered his mind and sense organs), well established in Self-Knowledge (atma-jnana). He says that "one who has mastered himself is always Self-satisfied, and he is free from all the desires. He is free from all worldly attachments and can enjoy true joyfulness. He is free from attachment, hatred, anger, fear and other mental disturbances. Even though they are living in the same world as the ignorant (ajnani), they can enjoy freedom and contentment. Krishna says "what is day for worldly people is night for Sthita-Prajna and what is night for worldly people is day for the Yogi". Worldly people seek happiness in material objects and are always trying to find the ways to attain them, while for a yogi all the material possessions are obstacles and he is searching for the Atman or Higher-self. (BG 2.55-57, 69)

Krishna says that our mundane mind is like the flooding rivers, breaking out of their banks, destroying all the fields, crops and whatever else comes in their path. While the higher mind or conscious mind of a yogi is like the ocean, where all the rivers can pour all their waters into them, the ocean not only takes the water but also never breaks the boundaries. The yogi or Self-realised mind is undisturbed from liking-disliking, pain-pleasure, and favorable-unfavorable. He uses the term Brahmi, one becomes one with the divine source. These yogis live like a jivan-mukta (liberated while living) and after death they become one with Brahman (Supreme Consciousness) and attain nirvana (liberation), which is known as Videha-mukta (free from birth cycles).

Arjuna's Enquiry, Samkhya Yoga

BG 2.1: Sanjay said: Seeing Arjun overtaken with pity, his mind suffering with grief, and his eyes full of tears, Lord Krishna spoke the following words.

BG 2.2: The Supreme Lord (Bhagavan) said: My dear Arjun, how has this delusion (moha) overcome you in this hour of peril? It is not appropriate for you as an honourable person. It does not lead you to the higher abodes of respect, but to disgrace.

BG 2.3: O Parth, this inhumane or unmanly spirit does not befit you at this point. Give up such petty weakness of heart and arise, O vanquisher of enemies.

BG 2.4: Arjun said: O Madhusudan, how can I shoot arrows in battle on men like Bhishma and Dronacharya, who are worthy of my worship, O destroyer of enemies?

BG 2.5: It would be better to live in this world by begging, than to enjoy all luxuries of life by killing these noble elders, who are my teachers. If we kill them, the wealth and pleasures we enjoy will be stained with their blood.

BG 2.6: We even do not know which result of this war is preferable for us—conquering them or being conquered by them. Even after killing them we will not desire to live. We know that they have taken the side of Dhritarasthra (Adharma), and now stand before us on the battlefield.

BG 2.7: I am confused about my duty and am overwhelmed with anxiety and faintheartedness. I surrender to you as your disciple, please guide me for sure as to what is best for me now.

BG 2.8: I am unable to find means of getting rid of this suffering and grief that is weakening my sensory abilities. Even if I win a flourishing and unparalleled kingdom on the earth, or gain authority like the celestial gods, I will be still unable to dispel this misery.

BG 2.9: Sanjay said: After saying all this, Gudakesh, that destroyer of enemies, addressed Hrishikesh: "Govind, I shall not fight," and remained silent.

BG 2.10: O Dhritarashtra, then, in the middle of both the armies, Lord Krishna smilingly spoke the following words to the grief-stricken Arjun.

BG 2.11: The Supreme Lord said: While you speak words of wisdom like a wise man (Jnani), you are grieving for that which is not worthy of grief. The wise grieve (Shauka) neither for the living (Jiva) nor for the dead (Mrita).

BG 2.12: There was not a time when I did not exist, nor you or all these kings and people. Also in future they shall never cease to exist.

BG 2.13: Just as the embodied soul uninterruptedly resides in this body from childhood to youth to old age, similarly, at the time of death, the soul moves to another body. The wise are not deceived by this.

BG 2.14: O son of Kunti, the contact between the senses and the sense objects gives rise to short-lived experiences of happiness and sadness (Sukha-Dukha). These are impermanent and arise and perish like the seasons of winter and summer. O descendent of Bharat, one must learn to face them without being disturbed and remain in balance (Samatva).

BG 2.15: O Arjun, finest amongst men, I know you are not affected by happiness and suffering, and one who is able to remain steady in both sukha-dukha, has attained eligibility for emancipation.

BG 2.16: All the materials which are subject to changes are impermanent, and of the atma or soul which is eternal there is no death. This has been perceived and detailed by the seers of the truth, after studying the nature of both.

BG 2.17: That which pervades this body, know it to be eternal. No one can cause any form of destruction or harm to the immortal soul.

BG 2.18: Only the physical body is perishable; the embodied soul that resides within the body is indestructible, immeasurable, and eternal. Therefore, fight, O descendent of Bharat.

BG 2.19: Neither of them holds the true wisdom —the one who thinks the soul can murder and the one who thinks the soul can be killed. For truly, the soul can never kill nor can it be killed.

BG 2.20: The soul has no birth, nor does it ever die; the soul simply exists and hence never ceases. The soul has no birth, it is eternal, immortal, and ageless. The soul is never destroyed even when the body is destroyed.

BG 2.21: O Parth, one who knows the soul to be immortal, eternal, unborn, and absolute, also knows that the soul cannot kill anyone or cause anyone to be killed.

BG 2.22: As a person changes worn-out clothes and wears new ones, likewise, at the time of death, the soul takes off its worn-out body and enters a new one.

BG 2.23: Weapons cannot tatter the soul, fire cannot burn it. Water cannot wet it, the wind cannot dry it.

BG 2.24: The soul is indestructible and incombustible; it can neither be moistened nor dried. It is eternal, all-pervading, unchangeable, absolute, and ancient.

BG 2.25: The soul is known to be invisible, inconceivable, and non-changeable. Knowing this, you should not grieve for the body.

BG 2.26: However, if you think that the self or atman is subject to birth and death, O mighty-armed Arjun, even then you should not grieve like this.

BG 2.27: Death is undeniable for one who has been born, and rebirth is unavoidable for one who has died. Therefore, you should not mourn over the inevitable.

BG 2.28: O successor of Bharat, all living beings (Jiva) are unmanifest before birth, manifest in life, and again unmanifest in death. So why do you grieve?

BG 2.29: Some see the soul as miraculous, some describe it as miraculous, and some hear of the soul as miraculous, while others, even on hearing, cannot recognise it at all.

BG 2.30: O Arjun, the soul that dwells within the body is immortal; therefore, you should not mourn for anyone.

BG 2.31: Also, consider your duty as a warrior, you should not hesitate. For a warrior, there is no better commitment than fighting for safeguarding of righteousness (dharma).

BG 2.32: O Parth, happy are the warriors to have such opportunities to defend righteousness, this is opening the doors and staircase to the celestial abodes for them.

BG 2.33: If you refuse to take part and fight in this righteous war (dharma-Yuddha), abandoning your social duty and reputation, you will certainly incur sin.

BG 2.34: People will speak of you as a coward and a fugitive. For a respectable person, dishonour is worse than death.

BG 2.35: The great warriors who hold you in high esteem will think that you fled from the battlefield out of fear, and thus you will lose their respect.

BG 2.36: Your enemies will defame and humiliate you with unkind words, disapproving your potency. Alas, nothing could be more painful than that.

BG 2.37: If you fight, if you are to be killed on the battlefield, you will go to the celestial abodes, or you will gain victory and enjoy the kingdom on earth. Therefore, arise with determination, O son of Kunti, and be prepared to fight.

BG 2.38: Fight for the sake of duty, treating equally happiness and distress, loss and gain, victory and defeat. Fulfilling your responsibility in this way, you will never incur sin.

BG 2.39: So far, I have explained to you Sāmkhya Yoga, regarding the nature of the soul. Now listen, O Parth, as I reveal Jnana Yoga, or the Yoga of Absolute Wisdom. When you work with such understanding, you will remain free from the bondage of karma.

BG 2.40: Living in this state of consciousness, there is no loss or adverse result, and even a little effort on this path saves one from great harm.

BG 2.41: O descendent of the Kurus, the intellect of those who are on this path is steadfast, and their goal is single pointed. But the intellect of those who are indecisive is multi-branched.

BG 2.42-43: Those with limited knowledge, get attracted to the fancy words of the Vedas, which advocate religious rituals for attaining to the celestial abodes, and belief in no higher principle is described in them. They glorify only those portions of the Vedas that please their senses, and perform self-important ritualistic ceremonies for attaining high birth, wealth, sensual enjoyment, and attainment to the heavenly planes.

BG 2.44: With their minds deeply attached to worldly pleasures and their intellects bemused by such things, they are unable to hold the firm determination for success on the path to Divine realisation.

BG 2.45: The Vedas deal with the three modes of material nature, O Arjun. Rise above the three modes to a state of eternal divine consciousness. Free yourself from dualities, and eternally keep firm in absolute truth, and without concern for material gain and safety, remain firm in the self.

BG 2.46: Whatever purpose is served by a small well of water is also naturally served in all respects by a large lake. Similarly, one who realises the Absolute Truth also fulfils the purpose of all the Vedic rituals.

BG 2.47: You have only the right to perform your given duties, but you have no control over the fruits of your actions. You are not the cause of the results of your activities, nor you are ever free from doing your Karma.

BG 2.48: Be firm and perform your duty, O Arjun, abandoning desires to succeed and fail. Such equanimity is called Yoga.

BG 2.49: Seek retreat in divine knowledge and discernment, O Arjun, and abandon fruit-seeking Karmas that are certainly inferior to Karmas performed with the wisdom found in Divine knowledge. Miserable are those who seek to enjoy the fruits of their actions.

BG 2.50: One who wisely practices the science of karma without attachment can attain freedom from both good and bad reactions in this life itself. Therefore, endeavour for Yoga, which is the art of skilful action, or being full of skill, awareness and conscience in all our actions and choices.

BG 2.51: The wise endowed with equanimity of intelligence (viveka), forsake attachment to the fruits of actions, which bind one to the cycle of life and death. By performing Karma in such consciousness, they attain the state beyond all suffering.

BG 2.52: When your intellect crosses the dilemma of delusion, you will then attain indifference to what has been heard and what is yet to be heard.

BG 2.53: When your intellect is freed from attraction towards the fruitive sections of the Vedic rituals and remains steadfast in divine consciousness, you will then attain the state of Siddha or perfect Yogi.

BG 2.54: Arjun said : O Keshav, what is the personality and qualities of one who is situated in divine consciousness? How does an enlightened person talk? How does he sit? How does he walk?

BG 2.55: The Supreme Lord said: O Parth, when one removes all selfish desires and cravings of the sensual desires that torment the mind, and remains established in the realisation of the self, such a person is said to be an absolute master or Siddha.

BG 2.56: One whose mind remains undisturbed among sorrow, who does not desire worldly pleasures, and who is free from attachment, fear, and anger, is known as a sage of steady wisdom (Sthita-Prajna).

BG 2.57: One who remains unattached in all situations and circumstances, and is neither delighted by good fortune nor dejected by misfortune, he is a Siddha with absolute knowledge.

BG 2.58: One who is able to withdraw the senses from their objects like a turtle withdraws its limbs into its shell when exposed to danger, is known as Siddha established in divine wisdom.

BG 2.59: Aspirants may restrain the senses from their objects of enjoyment, but the desire for the sensory objects remains as the nature of senses and mind. However, even these desires perish for those who realise the Supreme.

BG 2.60: The senses are so strong and tempestuous, O son of Kunti, that they can influentially carry away the mind even of a person endowed with discrimination and practicing self-control.

BG 2.61: They are established in absolute knowledge, who pacify their senses and keep their minds ever absorbed in ME (divine consciousness).

BG 2.62: While keeping the mind fixed and contemplating on the objects of the senses, one develops attachment to them. Attachment leads to desire, and from desire arises anger.

BG 2.63: Anger leads to the clouding of intelligence and discrimination, which results in disorientation of the memory. When the memory is disoriented, the intellect is destroyed; and when the intellect is destroyed, one is ruined.

BG 2.64: But one who controls the mind, and is free from attachment and aversion (Raga-Dwesha), even while using the objects of the senses, attains the Grace of Divine.

BG 2.65: By divine grace comes the peace in which all sorrows dissolve, and the intellect of such a person of tranquil mind soon becomes firmly established in the Divine.

BG 2.66: But an undisciplined person, who has no control of the mind and senses, can neither have a firm intellect nor steady focus and meditation on the Divine. For one who never unites the mind with the Divine there is no peace; and how can one who lacks peace ever be happy?

BG 2.67: Just as a strong wind sweeps a boat off its chartered course on the water, even one of the senses on which the mind focuses can lead the intellect into delusion.

BG 2.68: Therefore, one who has removed the senses from their objects, O well equipped and armed Arjun, is firmly established in true knowledge.

BG 2.69: What worldly beings consider as a day is the night of ignorance for the wise, and what all creatures see as night is the day for the self-absorbed sage.

BG 2.70: Just as the ocean remains in its limits and undisturbed by the never-ending flow of waters from rivers merging into it, likewise the sage who is firm or steadfast despite the exposer of desirable objects all around him attains peace, and not the person who strives to satisfy desires.

BG 2.71: The person, who renounces all material desires and lives free from a sense of greed, proprietorship, and egoism, attains absolute peace.

BG 2.72: O Parth, such is the state of an enlightened soul and he never again is deluded once he has attained it. Being founded in this consciousness even at the moment of death, one is liberated from the cycle of life and death and reaches the Supreme Abode of Divine.

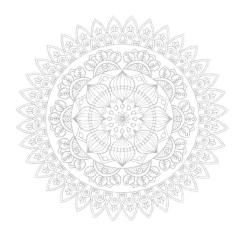

Chapter 3
Karma Yoga, Yoga of Action

In chapter 2, Krishna explains Samkhya, which is scientific knowledge of the Atman or Self known as atman-jnana or Self-Knowledge. Then further on he criticises religious activities and rituals based on myths for self-fulfilment (karma-kanda). Lastly, he explains about Karma Yoga.

This leads Arjuna into further confusion in deciding if he should fight or not. Arjuna says, "Divine Krishna, you are confusing me with your contradictory statements on Jnana and Karma, which both lead to moksha. Why would I not choose the path of Jnana Yoga instead of Karma Yoga, where I have to take part in this battle involving killings? (BG 3.1-2)

Krishna states that there are two paths or lifestyles one can chose to live - "Karma-yoga-Nistha (social life while doing all our duties) and Jnana-Yoga-Nistha (secluded life like a sage or monk, path of renunciation). One is the path of householders and the other is the path of monks. (BG 3.3) Krishna further says that whichever path one chooses, he or she has to still do the karma. He mentions that even contemplations, meditation for going inward for self-realisation, involve our Karma or actions. Of these two paths, Krishna advocates preference to social life throughout the Gita and encourages us to follow our dharma and fulfil all our duties. Further Krishna says to Arjuna that it is a sin not to follow your dharma. No one can live this life without doing some karma. If nothing else, you will breathe, eat, drink, sleep, think etc.

Krishna clearly mentions that doing your Karma is far better than not doing it. He said even if you do your Karma imperfectly, it will bring fruits, knowledge and experience. No one can attain purity, knowledge or self-realisation by abandoning their duties. A mind can never be left empty or unoccupied, it will be idle, and it will follow sensual-pleasure activities. He says by doing our duties (karma yoga) selflessly (niskama karma) one will attain Self-realisation. (BG 3.4-6)

Here lord Krishna classifies all our thoughts, feelings, emotions, desires, speech, eating, sleeping, sensory perceptions, physical actions etc. as Karma. So everything that we do at a mental, emotional, physical and spiritual level is all part of our Karma. This means we can never be free of doing Karma in life.

Further Krishna mentions that you must do your Karma like a Yajna- ceremony for invoking divine consciousness - so work becomes divine worship and it will lead us to self-realisation. If all our actions are driven by desires of material fulfilment, it will bring uncertainty, fear and mental disturbance. It will further cause attachment to worldly possessions, which leads us away from freedom and joyfulness.

Krishna says that if everyone will stop following their duties, this life cycle and Prakriti will come to end and hence we all must do our duties. Also, we must consider our life and everything that we have as a divine blessing, which will help purify our mind and senses.

Karma Yoga is necessary to maintain the harmony of the universe, which we are living in. We have an important role to play in this universal cycle of evolution and involution and we must fulfil our responsibilities (dharma and karma). (BG 3.14-16)
According to the teachings of Karma Yoga we can conclude that we must follow Karma Yoga as:

❏   It helps us grow materially and spiritually.
❏   Doing karma is to play our role in the universal evolution.
❏   It is our greatest offering to the Divine, serving society by fulfilling our duties.
❏   This brings and maintains harmony of our inner-self with the outer world (dharma).

Here in this chapter Krishna teaches us to follow niskama karma (fruitless or desireless Karma) and abandon Kamya-karma which is to fulfil our desires and sensual pleasures. A true yogi desires to perfect Niskama-Karma.

As before Krishna mentions that if we are alive, we are bound to take part in karma or actions. Like our senses are bound to perceive the fields of their experiences like smell for nose, sight for eyes, sound for ears, taste for tongue etc. But he says a Yogi doesn't allow the sense organs, mind and their actions to be uncontrolled. He keeps control and always remains mindful (sakshi) of all his actions and experiences. Karma Yoga ultimately leads one to liberation through use of viveka (reasoning, what is right and wrong to do), Suddhi (purity of body, mind and desires), vichara (contemplation and enquiry) and Jnana (Knowledge or wisdom of divine truth). Krishna uses the example of King Janaka who attained Jivan-Mukti (liberation while alive) and Atman-Jnana (Self-realisation) through his Karma-Yoga-Nishtha (faith and devotion in the yoga of action). (BG 3.17-20)

Further Krishna talks about the role of a wise man, yogi, or person of higher status (shrestha) in society (samaja). He says that these people have influence on others and many will follow you as an example. So if you don't do your Karma or fulfil your duties, others might take you as an example and that will cause further deterioration to society. He said in that case you will be responsible for all the negative outcomes. Hence fight this war not for your personal benefits but as your Kshatriya Dharma to establish peace and justice. (BG 3.21-25)

Krishna says that the wise must perform their duties to teach others while the ignorant must perform their duties to improve their skills and purify their intellect. (BG 3.27-29)

In the 30th verse in this chapter Lord Krishna states five conditions of Karma Yoga:
- ❏ Keep your mind focussed on self-realisation
- ❏ Offer all your actions to the divine cause or humanity
- ❏ Don't worry about or be attached to fruits or outcomes.
- ❏ Be free from desires and possessiveness.
- ❏ Maintain calmness and equanimity of mind.

Krishna says that one who follows their duties (karma yoga) and offers them to me (divine cause) will attain self-realisation and all true pleasures of life. Our likes (raga) and dislikes (dvesha) are born of vasanas (desires) and drive a man and his ego into habitual actions or unconscious actions and choices. We must do what needs to be done and not what we like to do or what we feel pleased in doing. (BG 3.31-35)

Arjuna asks here why human beings ever do the sinful or anti-social acts, causing harm, bringing injustice and suffering for others. Krishna says that the problem is rooted in Kaam (desires to please our senses) and raga-dvesha (liking and disliking). These are real enemies of a true seeker of spiritual realisation. When we don't get what we want, or things do not turn out the way we desire, we suffer with anger. Due to anger we lose our ability to think and use our intellect. This clouds our knowledge and wisdom. This further covers our Chetana or consciousness and we run after endless desires, which leads us away from peace and equanimity of mind. We must always keep awareness of senses, mind and the intellect as these are bases of lower mundane desires (phala-hetu-karma) or higher divine desires (niskama-karma). (BG 3.36-41)

We must replace Dur-vasanas (lower desires) by subha-vasanas (desires to benefit humanity or divine causes). All the false values should be replaced by moral and ethical values to bring love, peace and harmony through discrimination and reasoning (viveka and jnana). Through this righteous attitude and our righteous actions, kama will become weak, and our mind and senses will be purified, leading us to discover the Atma (atma-darshana). (BG 3.42-43)

Karma Yoga, Yoga of Action

BG 3.1-2: Arjun said: O Janardan, if you consider wisdom (Jnana) superior to action (Karma), then why do you ask me to take part in this terrible war? My intellect (buddhi) is puzzled by your confusing advice. Please tell me decisively the one path by which I may attain the supreme reality.

BG 3.3: The Divine Lord said: O sinless one, the two paths leading to self-realisation were previously explained by me: Jnana Yoga - the path of wisdom, for those inclined toward contemplation, and the path of work for those inclined toward action.
Here Krishna mentions two paths:
Antar Marga – Path of Jnana Yoga or contemplation where the sadhaka goes inward to attain self-realisation.

Bahira Marga – A path of Karma Yoga or Action where the sadhaka goes outward and performs all the duties selflessly to attain self-realisation.

BG 3.4: One cannot achieve freedom from karmic fruits or outcomes by merely abstaining from Karma, nor can one master wisdom by mere physical renunciation (Vairajna or Vairagya).

BG 3.5: No one who can ever remain without doing the Karma at any moment. Indeed, all beings are duty-bound to act by their qualities born of material nature (the three gunas of prakriti).

BG 3.6: Those who restrain the external organs of action (karmendriyas), while continuing to dwell on sense objects in their mind, certainly deceive themselves and are to be called hypocrites.

BG 3.7: But those karma yogis who control their senses of cognition (Jnanendriyas) with the mind, O Arjun, and engage the Karmendriyas (action senses) in Karma without attachment, are certainly superior.

BG 3.8: You should therefore perform your Vedic duties (dharma), since action (Karma) is superior to inaction (Akarma). By ceasing activity, even your physical body will not be sustained.

BG 3.9: Karma must be done as a yajña (sacrifice) to the Supreme Divine; otherwise, Karma will cause a burden in this material world. Therefore, O son of Kunti, perform your set of duties, without being attached to the fruits (Niskam Karma), for the attainment of Divinity.

BG 3.10: In the beginning of creation, Brahma created humankind along with assigned duties, and said, "Thrive in the performance of these yajñas (sacrifices), for they shall grant upon you all you wish to achieve."

BG 3.11: By your sacrifices the heavenly gods will be pleased, and by cooperation between humans and the heavenly gods, prosperity will flourish for all.

BG 3.12: The heavenly gods, being pleased by the performance of sacrifice, will bless you with all the necessities of life. But those who enjoy what is given to them, without making offerings in return, are verily robbers.

BG 3.13: The spiritually minded, who eat food that is first offered in sacrifice, are free from all kinds of sin. Others, who cook food for their own enjoyment, verily eat only sin.

BG 3.14: All living beings survive on food, and food is produced by rains. Rains come from the performance of sacrifice, and sacrifice is produced by the performance of fulfilling Dharma or assigned duties.

BG 3.15: The Dharma for human beings is described in the Vedas, and the Vedas are manifested by the Divine itself. Therefore, the all-pervading Divine is eternally present in acts of sacrifice (Yajna).

BG 3.16: O Parth, those who do not accept their responsibility in this cycle of sacrifice established by the Vedas are sinful. They live only for the satisfaction of their senses; indeed their lives are worthless.

BG 3.17: But those who rejoice in the Self, who are illumined and accomplished in the Self; for them there is no Karma.

BG 3.18: Such self-realised souls have nothing to gain or lose either in dismissing or renouncing their Karmas. Nor do they need to depend on other living beings to fulfil their self-interest or needs.

BG 3.19: Therefore, letting go of attachment, perform Karma as a subject of duty; by performing actions without being attached to the fruits, one attains the Supreme Divine.

BG 3.20-21: By performing their assigned duties, King Janak and others attained Siddhis or perfection. You should also perform your Karmas to set an example for the good of the world. Whatever Karmas great individuals perform, common people follow. Whatever standards they set, the rest of the world follows.

BG 3.22: There is nothing as Karma for me to do in all the three worlds, O Parth, nor do I have anything to gain or attain. Yet, I am engaged in performing my Karma.

BG 3.23: If I did not carefully perform the assigned Karma, O Parth, all men would follow my path in all respects.

BG 3.24: If I ceased to perform my Karmas, all these universes would perish. I would be responsible for the chaos that would triumph, and would thereby destroy the peace or balance of the human race.

BG 3.25: As ignorant people (Ajnani) perform their duties with the desires for the fruits, O offspring of Bharat, so should the wise (Jnani) act without attachment, for the sake of the welfare of the world (loka-sangraham).

BG 3.26: The wise should not create or fall prey or follow in the intellects of ignorant people, who are attached to fruits of their actions (phala-karma), by persuading them to stop actions. Rather, by performing their duties in a rational intellect manner (viveka-buddhi), they should inspire the ignorant also to do their Karmas.

BG 3.27: All actions are carried out by the three qualities (tri-gunas) of material nature. But in ignorance, the soul, deluded by false identification with the material world and body, believes itself to be the doer.

BG 3.28: O mighty-armed Arjun, an awakened person sees the soul as separate from gunas and karmas. They know that "it is only the gunas (in the shape of the body, senses, mind etc.) that interchange amongst the gunas (in the form of the objects of sensory experience), and thus they do not get entangled in them.

BG 3.29: Those who are deluded in this operation of the gunas become attached to the fruits of their actions. But the wise who know the truth should not disturb such ignorant people who know very little.

BG 3.30: Performing all Karmas as an offering unto me, always meditate on me as the Supreme Divine. They become free from desires and selfishness, and fight with letting go of your mental grief.

BG 3.31: Those who adhere by these teachings of mine, with insightful faith and free from whinge, are freed from the bondage of Karma.

BG 3.32: But those who find faults with my teachings, lacking of knowledge and devoid of discrimination, they disrespect these beliefs and lead to their own devastation.

BG 3.33: Even wise people act according to their natures, for all living beings are driven by their natural tendencies. What will one gain by suppression?

BG 3.34: The senses naturally experience attraction and aversion (raga and dwesha) to the objects of senses. Do not allow the self to be controlled by them, for they are hindrances and enemies.

BG 3.35: It is far better to perform one's own Duties or Dharma, though shaded with faults, than to perfectly perform duties or Karmas of others. In fact, it is superior to die in the performance of one's own duty, than to follow the path of another, which is burdened with peril.

BG 3.36: Arjun asked: O The descendent of Vrishni, "Why is a person driven to commit immoral acts, even unwillingly"?

BG 3.37: The Supreme Lord said: It is lust alone, which is born of contact with the mode of passion, and transformed into anger. Know this as the sinful, all-devouring enemy in the world.

BG 3.38: Just as a fire is covered by smoke, a mirror is masked by dust, and an embryo is concealed by the womb, similarly one's knowledge gets blanketed by desire.

BG 3.39: The wisdom or intellegence of even the most discerning wise ones gets covered by this unending enemy in the form of insatiable desire, which is never satisfied and burns like fire, O son of Kunti.

BG 3.40: The senses, mind, and intellect are said to be breeding grounds of desire. Through them, it clouds one's wisdom and deludes the embodied soul.

BG 3.41: Therefore, O best of the Bharatas, in the very beginning bring the senses and mind under control and eliminate this enemy known as desire, which is the embodiment of sin and devastates knowledge and realisation.

BG 3.42: The senses are superior to the gross body, and mind is superior to the senses. Beyond the mind is the intellect (buddhi), and even beyond the intellect is the soul (Atman).

BG 3.43: Thus, knowing the soul to be superior to the material intellect, O mighty armed Arjun, soothe the self (senses, mind and intellect) by the self (light of the soul), and eradicate this intimidating enemy called lust.

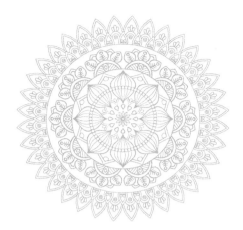

Chapter 4
Renunciation of Action; Jnana Karma Sanyasa Yoga

Lord Krishna explained Sankhya-Yoga and Karma-Yoga in the second and third chapters. These two Yogas are very well known from the beginning of the creation itself through the Karma-Kanda and Jñana-Kanda of the Vedas.

Krishna begins the fourth chapter by telling Arjuna that he initiated the lineage of Vivasvan (Lord Sun), Manu, Iksvaku, and others in the beginning of creation (through the Vedas). Krishna further says that "it is the same Vedic wisdom which is being revived by him to Arjuna in the form of the Gita because it has been forgotten by that time." (BG 4.2, 3).

Here, Arjuna asks Krishna, "How can he be the initiator of the ancient Vedic Wisdom (BG 4.4) while he is being born in same lifetime as him?" Krishna here explains about his Avataras (incarnations). He mentions that all living beings are born because of their own Karma (vyasti-karma) as well as the collective Karma of the world (samasti-karma). Krishna says that, "He does not have his own karma. But the karma of the world becomes the cause for the birth of the Divine."

The evil actions of the wicked and the noble worship of the saints necessitates the incarnation (avatara) of the Divine to punish the evil and protect the virtuous. Thus, the Divine incarnates to establish dharma in the universe (BG 4.7, 8).

Incarnation of the Divine takes place under his own Maya and hence the Divine's true nature is free from the cycles of birth, death and Karma and doesn't affects his nature of omni-science, omnipotence, etc. Krishna says that he remembers all the past incarnations, as well as His true nature while the rest of us have forgotten all of them.

Krishna says "I initiated the Vedic tradition." He further says that we all have existed eternally at each point and time, but we don't remember any of these births.

Krishna further explains his True Nature and its knowledge in the next few verses. Though the divine is active and exists in everything, He is still free from all activities (karma) and their fruits (phala) (BG. 4.13, 14).

He is akarta (no-doer) and abhokta (no-consumer). One who recognises this nature of the Divine also attains liberation i.e. becomes free from actions and their fruits (BG 4.9). This explains that the true nature of Atman or Jiva (soul, living being) and the Divine is one and the same.

Due to our attachment and interest in means and ends or actions and fruits, we lose this awareness of self or Purusha and its true nature. By freeing our mind from attachment, hatred, fear and greed as well as surrendering to the Divine, one attains Self-knowledge (atma-jnana). At this point of self-realisation the divine blesses the devotee or Bhakta with whatever they seek. (BG. 4.10,11)

In this chapter from the 16th to the 25th verse, Krishna explains the nature of action (karma) and inaction (akarma) and the characteristics of the person of such experience of the knower (Jnata). Here Krishna mentions that anything that is being done physically, mentally, verbally and spiritually is known as Karma or action which is being accumulated when done for desires and expectations of fruits. When the Karma is done without seeking or desiring for fruits it is known as Akarma and has no accumulation. Krishna further mentions that a "wise man is one who sees the Self free of all actions or doesn't have the attitude of 'I do' in activities performed by them". Here Sadhaka sees itself just as an instrument of divine purpose or action.

Our body continuously acts and functions to sustain all life process and can never fully relax as long as we are alive. As Krishna says, we can never be free of doing Karma. We are always doing something, if nothing else, we are still breathing, thinking, listening, sleeping or doing nothing - this also becomes action for the body. But we can relax and stay focused and live in equanimity at a mental and emotional level. This is the highest Jnana for renunciation of all our actions, seeing the Self as Drashta or observer and not doer or consumer.

The Jnani or wise man sees Brahma or the Divine behind and

in everything and nothing else (BG.4.25). Whether his body is active or doing something or not doing anything, he is doing any karma or not doing any karma, the Divine Self is unaffected by all this (BG. 4.20, 21).

The Self, Atman or Purusha is self-sufficient, contented, independent, equanimous, and free from expectations, desires, attachments, and jealousy and all forms of duality. His actions are devoted for the Divine purpose and benefits of humanity (BG. 4. 22, 23).

In the next few verses Krishna talks about how Jnana Yoga is the superior path of Sadhana compared to all other paths. He mentions that people without right knowledge will have no understanding of even what is true happiness, divine bliss and joy. Swamiji Dr Gitananda Giri Ji mentions this as "what is good may not be pleasant and what is pleasant may not be good for our Sadhana. So don't avoid good for sake of Pleasure". Hence Viveka, reasoning and right knowledge or wisdom becomes an important aspect of Sadhana. (BG. 4. 25 to 34).

This Jnana Yoga or true awareness of our true self, atma-jnana, known as Brahmajñana-yajña is the direct means to liberation. (BG.4. 33). To acquire and understand this atma-jnana or wisdom one should approach a Guru who has experienced this Truth (Tattva-darsshi) and who has the true knowledge and language to communicate it (jñani).

A Guru or teacher must be approached by seekers with humility, faith, reverence and true desire for this knowledge. Instructed by those Gurus or Masters through the scriptures and their experience, a follower or seeker also attains the atma-jnana or knowledge of self. (BG.4.34).

Acquiring this knowledge or wisdom, one will not be delusional again. At this point the Sadhaka or Jnani sees everything in the Divine and the Divine in everything as well as in himself or herself. Here we experience our identity with the divine and attain higher realisation of divinity as all-pervading (BG.4. 35). Through the means of a boat in this knowledge one crosses over the ocean of maya or illusion however vast it may be (BG.4. 36). Like a blazing fire burns everything and reduces to ashes, this knowledge burns and eliminate all the karmas (BG.4.37).

Hence, knowledge is the greatest and subtlest purifier. All other paths of sadhanas can produce punya, prana, and viriya which itself cab be a bondage without true knowledge. Jnana sadhana can eliminate ignorance which is the root cause of all our mental and emotional issues. That seeker who has purified the mind will soon attain this knowledge by the teaching of a guru (BG.4.38).

In the concluding verses in this chapter (verses 38 to 42), Lord Krishna talks about the qualifications (Yojnata) and disqualifications (ayojnata) of the seeker's Atma-Jnana or Self-knowledge.

Krishna says that, "One who has faith in the Guru and the shastra (scriptures and teachings), sense-control (atma-sanyam), and a sincere desire for self-realisation will gain the Self-knowledge (atma-jnana) (BG.4.39).

Further Krishna says, "one who is ignorant, faithless, and doubting this, he is lost in worldly sufferings. He has no joy or happiness in life (BG.4.40). Therefore, "Arjuna! Free yourselves from all these doubts regarding the validity of these spiritual quests, and follow the path of karma yoga (yoga of skill in action)", advises Lord Krishna (BC.4.42).

Krishna Mentions here that, "Karmas do not bind one who has mastered or known this Atma-Jnana or Self-Knowledge of soul as the eternal and divine being" (BC.4.42).

This is freedom through knowledge and performing our duties and actions (karma) with no desires of fruits -jñana-karma-sanyasa - is renouncing from all fruits of one's actions, and leads to absolute realisation.

Renunciation of Action; Jnana Karma Sanyasa Yoga

B.G. 4.1 The Supreme Lord said: I taught this eternal science of Yoga to the Sun-god (Surya), Vivaswan, who taught it on to Manu; and Manu in turn instructed it to Ikshvaku.

B.G. 4.2 O destroyer of enemies, the Adhikaris or eligible ones, received this science of Yoga in a continuous tradition or lineage (Paramparai). But over the long passage of time, it was lost to the worldly people.

B.G. 4.3 The same ancient eternal knowledge (Vidya) of Yoga, which is the supreme secrete, I am today revealing unto you, because you are my friend as well as my devotee, who can understand this transcendental knowledge.

B.G. 4.4 Arjun said: O Krishna, You were born in this modern time, which is much later to Vivasvan. I cannot comprehend that in the beginning you taught this science to Surya, the Sun God.

B.G. 4.5 The Supreme Lord said: Both you and I have had many births, O Arjun. You have forgotten them all, while I remember them all, O Paramtapa (one who has mastered the highest levels of Tapas).

B.G. 4.6 Although I am unborn, the Master or Divine Source of all living beings, and I am eternal nature, yet I appear in this world by quality of Yogamaya (my divine power).

B.G. 4.7 Whenever there is a decline in righteousness (Dharma) and an increase in unrighteousness (Adharma), O Arjun, at that time I incarnate (Avatar) myself on earth.

B.G. 4.8 To protect the righteousness or goodness (Dharma Raksha), to destroy the unrighteousness, and to re-establish the Dharma I appear on this earth, time after time (kaal).

B.G. 4.9 Those who realise the divine nature of my incarnation and activities or miracles (Lilas), O Arjun, upon leaving the body, they do not have to take birth again, instead they come to my eternal abode.

B.G. 4.10 Being free from attachment, fear, and anger, becoming well recognised in me, and taking refuge in me, many persons in the past became purified by knowledge of me, and thus they attained my divine love.

B.G. 4.11 In whatever way people surrender unto me, I respond with them accordingly. Everyone follows my path, knowingly or unknowingly, O son of Pritha.

B.G. 4.12 In this world, those who are desiring success in material activities worship the heavenly gods, with desires for material rewards to manifest quickly.

B.G. 4.13 The four classes (Varnas) of occupations were created by me according to people's qualities and rgw activities they perform. Although I am the creator of this system, know me to be the non-doer and eternal.

B.G. 4.14 Any Karma does not taint me, nor do I desire the fruits of action. One who knows me in this way is never bound by the karmic bondage of their Actions.

B.G. 4.15 Knowing this truth, even pursuers of emancipation in ancient times performed actions. Therefore, following the footsteps of those ancient sages, you too should perform your duty.

B.G. 4.16 What is action and what is inaction (Karma-Akarma)? Even the wise are confused in determining this. Now I shall explain to you the secret of Karma, by knowing which, you may free yourself from worldly bondage.

B.G. 4.17 You must understand the nature of all three— actions that need to be done (Karma), wrong action (Vikarma), and inaction (Akarma). The truth about these is insightful and challenging to understand.

B.G. 4.18 Those who know action in inaction and inaction in action are truly wise amongst humans. Although performing all kinds of actions, they are yogis and masters of all their actions. Knowing that the soul or Self is not the doer, all our actions or Karma becomes Akarma and free from any bondage. B.G. 4.19 The enlightened sages know those wise persons (Jnani), whose every action is free from the desire for material pleasures and who have removed or burned the seeds of Karma in the fire of divine knowledge.

B.G. 4.20 Such people, having given up desires to the fruits of their actions, are always fulfilled and not dependent on external things. Despite engaging in all the activities, they do nothing.

B.G. 4.21 People who are free from expectations and possessions, and disciplined in their mind and intellect, they encounter no sin, even though they are performing all their actions by means of the body.

B.G. 4.22. Content with whatever fruits they receive of their own accord, and free from jealousy, they are beyond the dualities of life (Dvandvas – liking or disliking, good or bad, pain pleasure). Remaining in equanimity (Samatva) in success and failure, they are not bound by their actions, even while performing all kinds of activities.

B.G. 4.23. They are liberated from the bondage of material attachments and their intellect is established in divine knowledge (Atma Jnana). Since they perform all Karma as a service or Dharma (to the Divine), they are freed from all Karmic consequences.

B.G. 4.24. For those who are well established in Divine Consciousness (Iswara), the oblation is Brahman, the server with which it is offered is Brahman, the act of offering is Brahman, and the sacrificial fire is also Brahman. Such persons, who view everything as Divine, easily attain HIM.

B.G. 4.25. Some religious people (Brahmins) worship the heavenly gods with material offerings unto them. Siddhas worship flawlessly who offer the Self as sacrifice in the fire of the Absolute Reality.

B.G. 4.26. Others offer hearing and other senses in the sacrificial fire of discipline or Tapas. While others offer sound and other objects of the senses as sacrifice in the fire of the senses (Pratyahara).

B.G. 4.27. Some, inspired by knowledge, offer the functions of all their senses and their life energy in the fire of the meditative mind (Dharna and Dhyana).

B.G. 4.28. Some offer their wealth as sacrifice, while others offer severe austerities as sacrifice. Some practice the eight-fold path of yoga (Ashtanga Yoga), and yet others study the scriptures and cultivate knowledge as sacrifice, while witnessing austere vows.

B.G. 4.29. 4.30. While others offer exhalation in the inhalation, some offer inhalation into the exhalation. Some laboriously practice Pranayama and restrain the incoming and outgoing breaths, purely absorbed in the regulation of the life-energy (Prana).

Yet others restrain their food intake and offer the breath into the life-energy as sacrifice. All these followers of sacrifice are cleansed of their impurities as a result of such performances.

B.G. 4.31. Those who know the secret of sacrifice, and are engaging in it, consume its leftovers that are like nectar, advance towards the Absolute Reality. O best of the Kurus, those who perform no sacrifice find no happiness either in this world or the subsequent.

B.G. 4.32. All these various types of sacrifice have been described in the Vedas. Know them as originating from different types of Karma; this understanding removes the knots of material bondage.

B.G. 4.33. O destroyer of enemies, sacrifice performed in knowledge is superior to any other material sacrifice. After all, O Parth, all sacrifices of Karma conclude in knowledge.

B.G. 4.34. Learn this Truth from a spiritual master (Sadguru). Inquire from him with devotion and selfless service unto him. Such an enlightened sage (Siddha) can disclose knowledge unto you because he has Experienced the Truth.

B.G. 4.35. Following this path and having achieved instruction from a Guru, O Arjun, you will no longer fall into delusion. In the light of that knowledge, you will see that all living beings are evolutes of the Supreme, and are within ME.

B.G. 4.36. Even those who are considered the most immoral of all sinners can cross over this ocean of mundane existence by sailing in the boat of Divine Knowledge.

B.G. 4.37. As a kindled fire reduces wood to ashes, O Arjun, so does the fire of knowledge burn all bonding of all Karmas to ashes.

B.G. 4.38. In this world, there is nothing as purifying as Divine Knowledge. One who has attained purity of mind through persistent Sadhana of Yoga, attains such knowledge within the heart, in due course of time.

B.G. 4.39. Those who possess deep faith and who have mastered their mind and senses attain divine knowledge. Through such transcendental knowledge, they quickly attain eternal supreme peace.

B.G. 4.40. But persons who hold neither faith nor knowledge, and who are of a doubting nature, suffer a downfall. For the sceptical souls, there is no happiness either in this world or the subsequent.

B.G. 4.41. O Arjun, actions do not bind those who have renounced Karma in the fire of Yoga, whose doubts have been dispelled by knowledge, and who are well established in knowledge of the Self.

B.G. 4.42. Therefore, with the sword of knowledge, distingush apart the doubts that have arisen in your heart. O offspring of Bharat, establish yourself in karma yoga. Arise, stand up, and do your Karma!

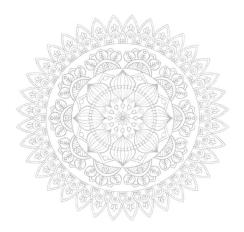

Chapter 5
Yoga of True Renunciation;
Karma Sanyasa Yoga

In Chapter 4 Lord Krishna explains Karma Yoga, renunciation and Yajna or ceremonial performances described in the Vedas and Yoga. He mentioned that a Jnani or person burns the bondage and seeds of karma in the fire of knowledge. A Jnani or wise man is free from all forms of possessions, and only performs Karma to sustain life. He is also happy with the fruits he receives as well as all the life events he faces (Prarabdha Karma). Krishna concludes the lesson by advising Arjuna to follow his duty.

Here we understand only two lifestyles known as Karma Marga (life of active action) and Sanyasa Marga (life of renunciation). The first is known as Karma Yoga and the second is known as Ashram-Sanyasa. In both the margas individuals are identified with the objects. Self is known as Samsari as it is identified as Karta or Doer. Neither of these Margas lead a Sadhaka to liberation. When Atma-Jnana or 'knowledge of self' is known and well established, one realises that he or she is 'Akarta', 'Abhokta and hence becomes 'Asamsari' or liberated one.

In a true sense, renouncing our identification with the body and sensory objects is true Sanyasa (renunciation) which is known as Jnana-Karma-Sanyasa. We can live our mundane life as a Sanyasi by renouncing the material desires and mental association with our actions and their fruits.

Ashram Sanyasa is totally renouncing the Karmic life or worldly life in the physical and mental sense. Krishna here advocates Jnana-Karma-Sanyasa to Arjuna and motivates him to take part in his Karma to fulfil his Dharma. We all seem to mistake the Sanyasa and Ashram Sanyasa as one or contradicting. Actually one leads into the other, sanyas or relinquishing the desire for the fruits of our actions will lead to a total renounciation where one will live apart from society rather in an ashram or solitude.

Chapter 5 begins with Arjuna's further confusion on how someone can take part in all their duties and also be a Sanyasi. Here Krishna reminds us that two Margas (Anter and Bahir or Jnana and Karma) are taking a Sadhaka to liberation by the means of Jnana Yoga. In both these paths, the Sadhaka needs to attain freedom from 'Raga-Dvesha' and become free of the two opposite dualistic natures. According to Krishna Karma Marga is more appropriate for a householder. He further mentions that a total renounced life is very difficult without appropriate training and discipline. (BG.5. 2 to 6)

A Karma Yogi dedicates all his physical, mental and spiritual actions to the divine without desiring or expecting any fruit. With this attitude of 'niskama-karma', all our actions become free of reactions in our mind. Gradually the sadhaka develops self-control and ultimately realises his True-Nature as the eternal Atman which is same in all beings. (BG.5. 7 to 12)

Further Krishna explains the characteristics and qualities of a Jnani or wise man and the highest wisdom. A Jnani knows his identity as the True Self and his nature is eternally the same as the True-Self. In the witnessing presence of the Self, all the faculties of body are functioning. The Self is not doing anything and neither does the Self initiate anyone to do anything. Actions are performed by the organs and instruments according to their nature and they reap the fruit accordingly. The Self is beyond good and evil in fruits. (BG.5. 13 to 21)

Many are deluded that they are doing everything and receiving the fruits because of delusion caused by ignorance (Avidya). When this ignorance of identifying the Self as doer and associating it with physical objects is removed, one attains the experience of the True Nature of Brahman. (BG.5. 15 to 16) A Jnani well established in the divine nature of Brahman through the Sadhana of Shravanam (listening to the truth), Mananam (contemplating the truth) and Nidhidhyasanam (meditating and becoming one with the Truth), the wise becomes one with the Brahman. Becoming free from all the impurities, the Sadhaka attains Videha-Mukti (free from body) and there is no more birth. A wise person sees one continuous awareness in all beings of existence and their functions. One overcomes mortality by recognising the identity with faultless, eternal, unchanging, all-pervading Brahman. Our Prarabdha (fruits of previous Karmas) brings favourable and unfavourable situations, but the wise remain unaffected in both and neither is excited nor depressed in those situations. One free from worldly associations and established in the Divine Nature of Brahman attains the Ananda (infinite true bliss). (BG.5. 17 to 21)

Unless a Sadhaka or seeker is detached from sensual pleasures, they cannot attain Ananda. A Viveka-Jnani (discriminative wise seeker) who knows the impermanence of sensory objects and the pleasures arising from them will not indulge in them. One who can restrain the impulses of Kama (desire) and Krodha (anger) alone is known as a man of self-control and eligible to enjoy life. (BG.5. 22 to 23)

Videha-Muktas or Jivan-Muktas are the ones who remain established in themselves, who are pure in their mind, who love all beings, and who have doubtless (nisandeha) knowledge of the Atman. (BG.5. 24 to 26)

In the last few verses Krishna gives a brief reference to meditation, which is discussed elaborately in the next chapter. This absolute knowledge can be attained by realising "I am not the body" and establishing our mind in "I am the divine".

Once the thoughts and mind are removed from the objects of the senses, the sense organs are withdrawn (Prahyahara), the breath regulated (Pranayama), and the mind is free from desires, fear and anger (Vairajna), one should meditate with a desire to attain Moksha. Such a Yogi becomes eternally liberated. Know the Divine is the receiver of all the sacrifices, He is the master of all worlds and whoever is the friend of all beings, Jnani or wise attains absolute peace and bliss known as Sat-Chita-Ananda. (BG.5. 27 to 29)

Yoga of True Renunciation; Karma Sanyasa Yoga

BG 5.1: Arjun said: O Shree Krishna, you have highly recommended karma sanyas (the path of renunciation of actions), and you also advocate tofollow karma yoga (selfless action with devotion). Please advise me decisively which of the two is more advantageous?

BG 5.2: The Supreme Bhagavan said: Both the path of karma sanyas and karma yoga lead to the supreme goal of liberation. But karma yoga is superior to karma sanyas.

BG 5.3: The karma yogis, who have no desire for anything as well as don't hate anything, are considered to be Sanyasi or renounced. Free from all dualities (liking-disliking, pain-pleasure etc), they are naturally liberated from the bonds of mundane cycles of cause and reaction.

BG 5.4: Only the ignorant (Ajnani) speak of sankhya, Karma Sanyasa and Karma Yoga as different. Jnanis or one who knows the Absolute reality knows that by following one of these paths, one attains the fruits of both.

BG 5.5: The Absolute State that is attained by means of karma sanyas is also attained by Karma Yoga. Hence, those who see karma sanyas and karma yoga to be identical, truly see the reality as it is.

BG 5.6: Absolute renunciation (karma sanyas) is difficult to follow or master without proper preparation through following Karma Yoga or action with devotion, O mighty-armed Arjun, but the sage who is skilled in karma yoga quickly attains the Supreme Reality.

BG 5.7: The karma yogis, who have purified their mind and intellect, and who practice discipline of the mind and senses, see the individual Self as the same in all beings. Though performing all kinds of actions, they are never caught in cause and reactions of Karma.

BG 5.8-9: Those who are firm in this karma yoga, always think, "I am not the doer," even while engaged in seeing, hearing, touching, smelling, moving, sleeping, breathing, speaking, excreting, and grasping, and opening or closing the eyes. With the light of divine knowledge, they see that it is only the material senses that are moving amongst their objects.

BG 5.10: Those who dedicate all their actions to the Divine purpose, forsaking all attachment, remain unaffected from all sins, just like a lotus petal is untouched by the mud beneath it.

BG 5.11: The yogis, while renouncing desires and attachment, perform actions with their body, senses, mind, and intellect, only for the purpose of self-purification.

BG 5.12: Offering the results of all activities to the Divine, the karma yogis attain eternal peace and joy (Ananda). Whereas those who are urged by their desires to perform actions with a selfish motive are entangled in Karmic bonding because they are attached to the fruits of their actions.

BG 5.13: While living in the body, those who are self-disciplined and detached dwell happily in the city of nine gates, free from thinking they are the doers or the cause of anything.

The Śhwetāśhvatar Upanishad:
navadwāre pure dehī hanso lelāyate bahi
vaśhī sarvasya lokasya sthāvarasya charasya cha   (3.18)

"The body consists of nine gates—two ears, one mouth, two nostrils, two eyes, the anus and genitals. In material consciousness, the soul residing within the body identifies itself with this city of nine gates. Within this body also resides the Supreme Consciousness, who is the master of all living beings in the world. When the soul establishes its connection with the Divine, it becomes free like Him, even while residing in the body."

BG 5.14: Neither the sense of 'I do' nor the nature of 'doing' or actions comes from the Divine; nor does He create the fruits of actions. All this is enacted by the modes of Gunas or qualities of material nature.

BG 5.15: The omnipresent Divine is not involved in the sinful or virtuous Karmas of anyone. The living beings are deluded because their true knowing of the Self is covered by ignorance.

BG 5.16: But for those in whom this ignorance of the self is purified by divine knowledge (atma-jnana), that knowledge reveals the Supreme Reality, just like the sun illumines everything in daytime.

BG 5.17: Those for whom the intellect is focused in the Divine, who are totally absorbed in the Divine, with firm faith in Him as the Supreme Goal, such Sadhakas soon reach the absolute state from which there is no return, and their sins are dispelled or removed by the light of knowledge.

BG 5.18: The truly knowledgeable, with the eyes of divine knowledge (Prajna Chakshu), see all beings with the equal vision (Sama-darshina) as in Brahmin, a cow, an elephant, a dog, and a dog-eater.

BG 5.19: Those whose minds are established in equality (sama-bhava) of vision overcome the cycle of birth and death in this very life. They possess the flawless qualities of the Divine, and are therefore contained in the Absolute Reality.

BG 5.20: Established in the Divine, having a firm understanding of divine knowledge and not being hindered by delusion, they neither rejoice in getting something favourable nor grieve when experiencing the unfavourable.

BG 5.21: Those who are not involved in the external sensory pleasures recognise divine bliss in the Self. Being united with the Divine through Yoga, they experience Ananda or eternal bliss.

BG 5.22: The pleasures that arise from contact with the objects of senses, though appearing as enjoyable to worldly-minded people, are verily a source of unhappiness. O son of Kunti, such pleasures have a beginning and an end, and so the wise do not delight in them.

BG 5.23: Those persons are known as Yogis, who are free from the forces of sensory desires (Kama) and anger (Krodha) before renouncing the body, and are living in absolute bliss or Anandam.

BG 5.24: Those who are happy within themselves, enjoying the bliss of Divine within, and are illumined by the inner light (antah-jyoti), such yogis are united with the divine (Brahma-Bhuta) and are liberated from the material reality (Brahma-Nirvanam).

BG 5.25: Those saintly persons (Rishis), whose sins have been eliminated, whose doubts are removed, whose minds are disciplined, and who are devoted to the welfare of all beings, attain the Divine and are liberated from material existence.

BG 5.26: For those sanyasis, who have freed themselves from anger and lust through continual determination, who have quietened their mind, and are self-realised, liberation from material existence is both here in life and hereafter the life.

BG 5.27-28: Quietening the mind and/or removing all thoughts of external enjoyment, with the mind's gaze fixed on the space between the eyebrows (Bhru-Madhya), balancing the flow of inhalation and exhalation in the nostrils, and thus mastering the senses, mind, and intellect, the sage who becomes free from desire and fear, always lives in freedom (Jivan-Mukta).

BG 5.29: Having realised Me as the receiver of all sacrifices and austerities, the Supreme Divine of all the worlds and the selfless Friend of all living beings, My devotee attains absolute peace (Shanti).

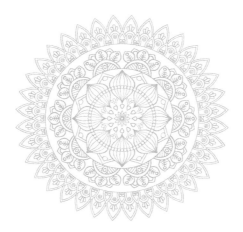

Chapter 6
Yoga of Meditation; Dhyana Yoga

Lord Krishna in chapter 6 teaches us the concepts of meditation or Dhyana as a path to liberation. The key idea is to focus our mind on the Individual Self (Purusha) and Divine Self (Parmatman) to attain Atma-Jnana or self-realisation. This will actually lead us to experience the teachings and wisdom we are blessed to receive from our Guru or teacher. The only way to be free of our natural conditioning of "I am the body or I do everything" is to become mindful through our own experience or Self-Knowledge.

Key ideas to learn in this chapter:
1.   Bahiranga-sadhana—following the Karma, Hatha Yoga and Jnana Yoga in daily life, which will lead to meditation or stillness of mind.
2.   Antaranga-sadhana — Following inner practices of Pratyahara and Dharna leading us to meditation.

3.   Dhyana-swarupam — Nature and types of meditation.
4.   Dhyana-phalam — Fruits of meditation.
5.   Dhyana-pratibandha-pariharau — Obstacles on the path of meditation and their remedy.

Few Key Terms:-
Manas or Mind: The field of thoughts and perception.
Buddhi or Intellect: The field of analysis, decisions and viewpoints.
Chitta or mundane mind: When Manas or the subtle mind is attached to an object or person.
Ahamkara or Ego: When the 'I' identifies with the material world and becomes proud of things like wealth, status, beauty, and learning, we call it ahankar, or ego.

Bahiranga Sadhana
Karma Yoga as a path to live our life at its optimum potential with discriminative knowledge (Viveka-Jnana) and free from desires for fruits naturally leads one to master self-control (Atma-Sanyam). It transforms the destructive extrovert mind into a contemplative and reflective single-pointed or Ekagra mind. Once we master our life and mind, we should aim to live a quieter life as a busy and over sensory stimulated life is an obstacle on the path of meditation. Further we should aim to develop total detachment from sensory objects and desires to enhance our contemplative and meditative abilities.
Two key practices for Karma Yogis are:

1.   Self Confidence (Atma-Vishwas): trusting our individual self to develop the willingness to follow the path and achieve success.

2.   Self-Control (Atma-Sanyam): self-discipline to follow
        the straight virtuous path of Karma.

Krishna mentions that one who lacks these two, become his or
her own obstacle to achieve success in any goal of life. While
the one who enjoys self-confidence and self-control finds
himself or herself to be enriched through their own right-use-
nes of energy, self sustaining and conserving energetically in
every field of life. Through this he soon attains the vision or
experience of the Atma-Anubhuti or vision of equality of soul
in each being.

For the Sadhaka following the Bahiranga Path, moderation
is also important. Moderation in eating, sleeping, working,
resting, talking, reading etc is the way to attain success in
Sadhana.

Antaranga Sadhana

In the second part Lord Krishna explains how to prepare a
space, seat, posture and mind followed by an explanation
of Dharna or a concentration technique. A Dhyana Sadhaka
needs to choose a clean and peaceful place, and find a
seat which is not too low on the ground nor too high, and
not too soft neither too hard. One should hold an erect and
comfortable posture with the body, neck and head held in
a straight, upright position. Further fix your mind at the tip
of the nose with the eyes half open. Next withdraw the mind
and sense organs from all the external activities and focus
your mind on your harmonious breathing. Once your mind is
calm, stable, clear and single-pointed, focus your mind on the
Parmatman or Divine Consciousness. (B.G. 6. 10-14)

Dhyana Swarupam and Phalam

Dhyana or meditation is a state of mind being absorbed in the Self or Atman. Once one has withdrawn the mind from sensory objects, one should use Viveka Jnana (discriminative intellect) to get rid of all the desires and attachments and pay attention to the absolute reality of Atman and there should be no other thought. The mind may get distracted, but a sincere Sadhaka with his mindful effort should keep bringing the mind again and again back to the Divine Consciousness or Truth.

According to Vedanta all and everything, including our thoughts, are just the mere objects of the Atma, or the Eternal Awareness. The Atma is not the object, thought, body, senses, or experience. Atma is the Absolute self 'I'. The highest form of meditation is "focusing our mind on I am divine – Aham Brahmasmi', or 'Soham – I am eternal consciousness'.

By continually focussing the mind on the Atma, the Sadhaka attains a state of absolute bliss and peace and reaches the state of liberation in this life only (Videha-mukti). In this state, the Sadhaka enjoys the pure state of peaceful mind, the one fully content in realisation and oneness with the Atman. Ananda or absolute bliss is not subject to sensual experience, it is transcendental in nature, which has no limits. Once realising the state of wholesomeness, and perfection, the Sadhaka never loses the sight of his True Nature. (B.G. 6. 20-28)

In this state of Ananda, he feels no excitement in even the greatest of favourable gains and doesn't lose his inner peace even when experiencing the greatest of losses. This absolute state of Ananda can never be lost as it was never gained. It is eternally there, we need to simply experience it. It is revealed by removing the false association that "I am suffering". The process of meditation is more to dissociate our mind from suffering and pain, which is known as Jivan-Mukti.

In this living meditation, a Sadhaka sees the Atman in all beings and all beings in Atma and remains established in this sense of oneness and equality. This knowing of Atma is also a knowing of the Parmatman or divine as they are not different. Even though a Dhyana Sadhaka is still performing all the Karmas, but remains established in divine Atma. Knowing the Atma, one sees everything. including their own body, with the attitude of non-possessiveness. He becomes free from selfish desires and effortlessly established in Dharma and is known to be a Saint. (B.G. 6. 29-32)

Dhyana Pratibandha Pariharau

Here Arjuna mentions that it is not easy to keep the mind focussed as it is naturally drawn to sensory objects and thoughts which are understood to obstacles in meditation. Our mundane mind by its nature seems to be restless and extrovert. This nature of mind makes it difficult to meditate and keep the mind focussed on the Atma. The frustrated mind of Arjuna enquires of Krishna regarding solutions. (B.G. 6. 33-34)

Krishna explains that "Abhyasa or practice and Vairajna or dissociation" are two solutions. Our mind is extrovert because it is attached with the desires and sensory objects. Removing the mind away from the desires and sensory experiences is Vairajna. Also due to our past experiences, memories, habits and Samaskaras, our mind also becomes restless. This has to be gradually removed by continual effort, practice and letting go. This is Abhyasa or practice. This also requires mental discipline, determination and patience. (B.G. 6. 35-36)

Arjuna so far believes that liberation is not possible in one life and hence asks Krishna, "what happens to that seeker who has fallen off or deviated from the Path of Self-realisation? Does he perish just like the scattered cloud?" As it was mentioned earlier how such people who focus their mind on the divine accumulate no Karma, Arjuna is not sure if these seekers have failed to achieve liberation and have gained nothing. Do these seekers suffer the consequences of deviating from the path of Punya and Moksha? Arjuna requests Krishna for clarification. (B.G. 6. 37-39)

Krishna states that "a spiritual seeker, even if they deviate from the path, can never have committed sin in doing their Sadhana". Meditation is a Punya-Karma capable of leading the Sadhaka to a heavenly experience and an ideal birth for the next life in order to continue their spiritual journey. A Yoga-Bhrasta (one who has deviated from the Yoga Path) is reborn in a well-cultured, prosperous family with the ideal opportunity for further growth. (B.G. 6. 41-42)

Being born in such an ideal situation, one will easily learn the wisdom they obtained from their previous life. Due to the nature of our Karma to carry the past Samaskaras, he will find his spiritual quest easily and without much effort this flame or light of wisdom will soon grow. Our previous Samaskaras will support the spiritual path to fulfil the ultimate life mission of self-realisation. (B.G. 6. 43-45)

Yoga of Meditation; Dhyana Yoga

BG 6.1: The Divine Lord said: Those who perform their assigned Karmas without desiring for the fruits of their actions are actual Sanyasis (renounced ones) and Yogis, not those who have merely been busy in performing sacrifices such as Agni-Hotra Yajna or abandoned physical activities.

BG 6.2: What is known as Sanysa is not different to Yoga, for no one can become a Yogi without renouncing material desires.

BG 6.3: To the Self who is aspiring to master Yoga, performing Karma without attachment is known to be the means and the path; to the sage who is already established in Yoga, attaining tranquility through practicing meditation is said to be the path and means.

BG 6.4: When the Sadhaka is not attached to the objects of the senses or to the actions themselves, that person is known to have mastered the science of Yoga. This is attained by means of renouncing all desires for the fruits of actions.

BG 6.5: Awake and raise yourself up by using the power of your mind, and not allowing yourself to . Your mind can be the friend and also the enemy of the self.

BG 6.6: The mind is the best friend for those who have mastered it. The mind is the worst enemy for those are being controlled by the mundane mind.

BG 6.7: The Yogis who have mastered the mind attain freedom from the dualities of hot and cold, pain and pleasure, disrespect and respect. Such Yogis remain peaceful and steadfast in their Bhakti (devotion to the Divine).

BG 6.8: The Yogis who are deeply content in knowledge and discernment and have transcended their senses, remain undisturbed in all situations. They perceive everything—dirt, stones, and gold—as the same and equal.

BG 6.9: The yogis look upon all—friends, families, enemies, the virtuous, and the sinners—with an unbiased intellect. The Yogi who has equinimity towards friend, companion, and foe, neutral among enemies and relatives, and impartial between the righteous and sinful, is considered to be renowned among humans.

BG 6.10: Those who are seeking to attain the state of Yoga should live in solitude, continually engaged in meditation with a skilful mind and body, letting go of desires and pleasurable possessions.

BG 6.11: To practice Yoga, one should make an asana (seat) in a dedicated place, by placing kusha-grass, deer skin, and a cloth, one on top of the other. The asana should be neither too high nor too low.

BG 6.12-13: Seated firmly on it, the Yogi should endeavour to purify the mind by focusing it in meditation with single-pointed focus, controlling all thoughts and activities. He should hold the body, neck, and head firmly in an erect position with ease, and gaze the eyes at the tip of the nose, without allowing the sight to wander and keeping the eyes half open and half closed.

BG 6.14: Thus, with a tranquil, fearless, and steadfast mind, and faithful in the vow of Brahmachariya, the watchful Yogi should meditate on ME (Parmatman), having me alone as the supreme goal to attain.

BG 6.15: Thus, continually keeping the mind absorbed in me, the Yogi of disciplined mind attains nirvan or liberation, and dwells in ME in supreme peace (Shanti).

BG 6.16: O Arjun, there is no success in Yoga for those who eat too much or do not eat enough, sleep too much or do not sleep enough, do too much or do not do enough.

BG 6.17: But those who are moderate in eating and lifestyle or daily life patterns (Jiva-Vritti), sensible in actions, and measured in sleep, can attain freedom from all sorrows by practicing Yoga.

BG 6.18: With comprehensive discipline, they master withdrawing the mind from selfish longings and transcend them to reach the divine eternal goodness of the Self. Such people are known to be in Yoga, and are free from all desires of the sensory objects.

BG 6.19: Just like the flame of a lamp in a place free from the blowing wind remains free from flicker, so the self-controlled mind of a Yogi remains steady in meditation on the Self.

BG 6.20: When the mind is dissociated from material activities, and attains stillness by the practice of Yoga, then the Yogi is able to witness the Soul through the refined mind, and he rejoices in the inner joy of Satchitananda.

BG 6.21: In that blissful state of Yoga, known as samadhi, one experiences absolute infinite divine bliss – Satchitananda - and thus established in that, one never deviates from the Eternal Truth.

BG 6.22: Having attained that state, one does not consider any accomplishment to be greater than that. Being thus self-realised, one is not troubled even in the middle of the greatest catastrophe.

BG 6.23: That state of detachment from union with despair and suffering is known as Yoga. This Yoga should be practiced with determination, free from hopelessness and negativity.

BG 6.24-25: Absolutely renouncing all desires arising from the worldly thoughts, one should discipline the senses from all sides with the conscious mind. Gradually and progressively, with faith in the intellect, the mind will merge into the Divine alone, and will think of nothing else.

BG 6.26: Whenever and wherever one finds the mind restless, unsteady wandering, one should bring it back and continually focus it on Divine.

BG 6.27: Great transcendental joy and peace (prashanta) is experienced by the Yogi with the calm mind, whose wordly passions are transcended, who is free from wrongdoing, and who sees everything in association with the Divine.

BG 6.28: A Yogi mastered in self-control unites the Self with Supreme Self, becomes free from worldly impurity, and, remaining in continual connection with the Supreme, achieves the highest state of absolute bliss known as Ananda.

BG 6.29: The true Yogis, uniting their consciousness with the Divine Consciousness, perceive it all with equal vision (Sam-Drishti) as "all living beings in Divine and Divine in all living beings".

BG 6.30: For those who perceive me universally and see all things in me, I am never lost to them, nor are they ever lost to me.

BG 6.31: A Yogi who is established in union with me, and devoted to me as the Supreme Soul residing in all beings, dwells only in me, though engaged in all kinds of worldly activities.

BG 6.32: I see them to be perfect Yogis (Yoga Siddha) who see the true equality of all living beings and respond to the joys and sorrows of others as if they were their own.

BG 6.33: Arjun said: The Yoga that you have described to me, O Madhusudan, appears impractical and unachievable to me, due to the restless nature of the mind.

BG 6.34: O Krishna, the mind seems to be always restless, turbulent, strong and stubborn. It looks to me that it is more difficult to control the mind than the wind.

BG 6.35: Lord Krishna said: O mighty-armed son of Kunti, what you say is accurate; the mind is indeed very difficult to contain. But by practice (Abhyasa) and detachment (Vairajna), it can be mastered.

abhyasa vairagyabhyam tannirodha (Yoga Darshan 1.12)

"The whirlpools of the mind can be mastered by continuous practice and detachment."

BG 6.36: Yoga is difficult to attain for one whose mind is uncontrolled. However, those who have learnt to govern their mind, and who strive sincerely by the appropriate means, can attain perfection in Yoga in my opinion.

BG 6.37: Arjun said: What happens to the Sadhakas who are not successful in their goal to attain Self-Realisation; one who begins the journey with faith, but who does not endeavour due to an unstable mind, and is unable to reach the goal of Yoga in this life?

BG 6.38: O mighty Armed Krishna - Do such people who deviate from Yoga get deprived of both material and spiritual success and perish like a scattered cloud in the sky?

BG 6.39: O Krishna, please dispel this doubt of mine completely, who other than you can do so?

BG 6.40: The Supreme Lord said: O Parth, One who participates on the spiritual path does not perish either in this world or the other worlds. My dear friend, one who attempts to achieve Divine-realisation is never overcome by evil.

BG 6.41-42: The Yogis deviated from the path reach the abodes of the virtuous upon death. After residing there for a long period of time, they are again reborn in the earthly plane, into a family of virtuous and flourishing people. They will be born into a family established in divine spiritual wisdom after death, if they had developed dispassion due to long practice of Yoga. Such a birth is very difficult to attain in this world.

BG 6.43: On taking such a birth, O descendant of Kurus, they will reawaken the wisdom of their previous lives, and strive with even firmer resolution towards mastering Yoga.

BG 6.44: Indeed, they feel naturally drawn towards the Divine, even against their own will, on the strength of their past Samaskaras. Such seekers naturally rise above the ritualistic ideologies of the scriptures.

BG 6.45: With the accumulated qualities of many past lives, when these Yogis engage in sincere endeavour for making further progress, they become purified from material desires and attain perfection in this life itself.

BG 6.46: A Yogi is superior to the tapasvi (ascetic), superior to the jnani, and even superior to the karmi (ritualistic performer like Brahmins). Therefore, O Arjun, strive to be a Yogi.

BG 6.47: Of all Yogis, those whose minds are always absorbed in me, and who engage with me with great devotion, I consider them to be the highest of all.

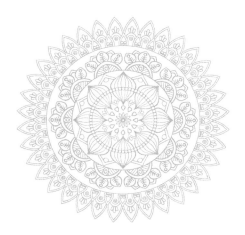

Chapter 7
Knowledge and Wisdom;
Jnana Vijnana Yoga

In the first 6 chapters, Krishna has explained to us the nature of the Individual Self, Karma Yoga, Selfless Attitude, Sanyasa and Dhyana Yoga. From Chapter 7 Krishna explains the nature of the Divine, Bhakti Marga or path of devotion and attributes (Upasana) etc. So far, we have been contemplating and working on our individual effort or Sadhana. The next step is to understand how the divine plays its role and blesses us on this spiritual path of selfless Karma and Yoga.

One who worships the Divine and surrenders the Self to the divine with the form or attributes, and qualities known as and by Siddhas, will ultimately attain union with the formless or the attribute-less Divine. Knowing the Divine or Parmatman as different to the individual Self or Atman is Jnana and knowing of the self and divine as one is known as Vijnanam. Vijnana is the highest knowledge and absolute Truth, which fulfils the intellectual quest of the Seeker.

Krishna mentions that the number of people who seek for this absolute wisdom is rare. Out of those only a few succeed on this path of Divine Realisation. (B.G. 7. 1-3)

Krishna mentions that the Divine has the lower nature (apara-prakriti – the field of manifested world) and the highest nature (para-prakriti- unmanifest eternal cosmic consciousness). The lower nature has eight divisions: - five major elements (pancha-mahabhutas), cosmic ego, cosmic intellect and the unmanifest potential. This is known as lower due to being subject to change, inert, limited and dependent. Higher nature is consciousness which is eternal in nature. This is behind all material bodies and sustains the entire universe. Para-Prakriti is not subject to change and it is conscious, infinite, and independent in nature and existence. In this concept, the divine is all that exists in a true sense and consists of conscious and manifest aspects known as Jiva and Jagat. The Divine alone creates, sustains and dissolves the universe. From the divine perspective there is no creation and the Divine Self alone is the very essence of all and everything. The Divine is the material cause of everything and hence everything is dependent upon Him but the divine is independent of everything. (B.G. 7. 4-12)

The worldly suffering (Samsara) is caused by the delusion of understanding the ultimate reality to be material creation, which is the product of the Tri-Gunas of apara-prakriti. This doesn't allow us to know the higher or ultimate nature or para-prakriti of the Divine Consciousness. We all are caught in what we see and experience. If we are satisfied in seeing the god in a statue, we will never seek any further. The Divine is behind each and every creation, but not the material object itself; the Divine takes in all beings or is behind all the aspects of creation, but not the actual objects.

Overcoming this illusion (Maya) consisting of the three Gunas is merely not possible by one's own effort. This crossing of endless maya is possible by "surrendering to the Divine Consciousness". (B.G. 7. 14)

Krishna classifies human living beings in five groups based on the belief systems, mindset and lifestyle. Lowest of them are the ones who don't believe or accept the Divine as the Supreme Consciousness. These people live their life governed by their own desires and are completely lost in the material world of illusion or maya. Others believe in the Divine and they are Bhaktas or devotees and worship or follow the divine in different forms, attributes and levels of maturity. The Artha are the ones who worship the divine only when they are suffering in life. The Artharthi worship the divine for the material fruits of health and prosperity. Jijnasu are the ones that have the ability to see the limitation of all material existence and seek the divine through wisdom or viveka. A Jnani is one who has attained absolute realisation and oneness with the Divine. (B.G. 7. 15-16)

Devotion of a Jnani is continual and well-established. A Jnani loves the divine as he loves himself as he sees no distinction between the two (advaita or non-dualism). The Divine loves such people as Himself. The Divine blesses such people with his divine formless non-dual vision. One can attain such vision through many births and divine blessing. (B.G. 7. 17-19)

Artharthis worship the divine for fulfilment of their desires for short-lived material fruits. They seek for divine blessings in the form of health, wealth, power, pride etc. and seek for those fruits by means of rituals and vows (vrita). The Divine, out of compassion, fulfils these prayers for those seekers. Anything other than Divine Realisation or Oneness is limited and changeable. (B.G. 7. 20-23)

The Divine reveals His true nature as being identical with the Sadhakas' natures and gained knowledge (of Prakriti and Jnana). The Divine is ever evident, imperishable, supreme, incomparable, and unborn. People deluded by maya mistake the Divine as the person or form subject to the birth, attributes, qualities etc. The Divine is non-dual (Advaita) in nature and knows everything from the past, present and future. The Divine is not even the object of knowledge or Jnana. (B.G. 7. 24-26)

Due to the fundamental self-ignorance no one can avoid the desires and illusion or maya in the initial stages of life. Naturally we go through the phases of Arta and Artharthi. Through worship, devotion and following the path of Karma Yoga, a seeker's mind is purified and gradually becomes desireless. He becomes Jijnasu. At that point a Sadhaka's attention naturally moves inward to seek for true knowledge and bliss, endeavouring for Absolute Self-Realisation. Soon he becomes a Jnani or master of Bhrahma, Karma, Adhyatma, Adibhuta, adidaiva and adiyajna. He knows para-prakriti and apara-prakriti as aspects of the Divine. Being established in such wisdom, he would not lose sight of the divine even at the moment of death. Thus the Jnani-Bhakta attains both the states of Jivanmukti and Videhamukti. (B.G. 7. 27-30)

Knowledge and Wisdom;
Jnana Vijnana Yoga

BG 7.1: The Shree Bhagawan said: Now listen, O Arjun, now, with the mind devoted exclusively to me, you can free all your doubts and know me completely by surrendering to me through the practice of Bhakti yoga.

BG 7.2: I shall now disclose unto you fully this knowledge and wisdom, after knowing which nothing else remains to be known in this world.

bhakti-yogena manasi samyak praihite 'male
apaśhyat puruha pūrva māyā cha tad-apāśhrayām
(Bhagavatam 1.7.4)

"Through bhakti-yoga, Ved Vyas established his mind upon the Divine without seeking for any material fruits, and thus attained the complete vision and realisation of the Supreme Divine Personality along with His external energy, Maya, which was under His control."

BG 7.3: Amongst many thousands of people, only one attempts for the perfection; and amongst those who have attained perfection, only very few realise this ultimate truth.

BG 7.4: Earth, water, fire, air, space, mind, intellect, and ego are the material evolutes or manifests of my divine energy.

tasmadvā etasmādātmana ākāśhah sambhūtah
ākāśhādvāyuh vāyoragnih agnerāpah
adbhyah prithivī prithivyā aushadhayah
aushadhībhyo 'nnam annātpurushah
sa vā esha purusho 'nnarasamayah   (Taittirīya Upanishad 2.1.2)

The material energy in its primordial form is known as prakriti. The Divine glimpses at it when He wishes to create the Universe. His shine stirs and creates mahān (this is the subtlest and potential energy from which each and everything manifests). Mahān further manifests into ahankār. Ahankār, in turn, gives rise to the pañch-tanmātrās or the five perceptions of – taste, touch, smell, sight, and sound. These tanmatras give birth to the five major elements— space, air, fire, water, and earth.

BG 7.5: Such is my manifested energy. But beyond it, O mighty-armed Arjun, I have an unmanifest and eternal energy. This is the jiva shakti (the conscious energy), which involves the individual souls who are the basis of life in this world.

"There are three states of existence: 1) Matter, which is changeable 2) The individual soul, which is eternal and unchangeable 3) Divine Consciousness, which is all pervading (matter and souls). By meditating upon the Divine, uniting with Him, and becoming one with Him, the soul is freed from the worldly illusion (samasarik maya)." (Shwetashvatar Upanishad 1.10)

"Just like the sun dwells in one place but its sunlight permeates the entire solar system, similarly there is One Divine, who by His infinite and boundless powers pervades the three worlds." (Vishnu Puran 1.22.53)

BG 7.6: Know that all living beings are manifested by these two energies of mine. I am the source of the entire creation, and it dissolves back into me.

BG 7.7: I am the Supreme One and there is nothing higher than

Me, O Arjun. Everything is bound and rests in me, as beads are wound on a thread in a Mala.

"There is nothing equal to the Divine, nor is there anything superior to Him." (6.8 Shwetashvatar Upanishad)

BG 7.8: I am the flavour in water, O son of Kunti, and the luminosity of the sun and the moon. I am the sacred syllable Om in the Vedic mantras; I am the sound in Akash, and the potential in humans.

BG 7.9: I am the primordial aroma of the Earth, and the brilliance and heat in the fire. I am the life-force in all beings, and the penance (Tapas) of the ascetics (Tapasvi).

BG 7.10: O Arjun, know that I am the eternal seed of all beings. I am the intellect of the intelligent, and the splendour of the glorious.

BG 7.11: O best of the Bharatas, I am the strength of a strong person. I am the virtue in people established in dharma free from Kama (sensual desires) and Raga (passion and attachment).

BG 7.12: The three states of material existence and qualities— Sattva or purity, Rajas or action, and Tamas or inertia—are manifested by my energy. They are in Me, but I am beyond them.

BG 7.13: Deluded by the three modes of Maya, the people caught in this material world are unable to know Me, the immortal and eternal.

BG 7.14: It is very difficult to overcome My divine energy Maya of Tri-Gunas or three primordial qualities of Prakriti. But those who surrender unto Me overcome this easily.

"Maya is the energy (prakriti), while God is the Essence of the energy." (Shwetashvatar Upanishad 4.10)
"Some people think Maya is mithyā (non-existent), but in reality Maya is an energy engaged in the service of the Divine in Creation, Preservation and Dissolution." (The Ramayana)

BG 7.15: Four kinds of people do not surrender unto me:

1. Those who are ignorant of divine knowledge (Mudha)
2. Those who are lazy and caught in their lower nature
3. Those who are deluded in their intellect
4. Those with a demoniac nature.

BG 7.16: O best amongst the Bharatas, four natures of virtuous people participate in my devotion—the distressed (artah), the seekers of worldly pleasures and possessions (artharthi), seekers pf knowledge (Jnanarthi), and those who are well established in knowledge (Jnani).

BG 7.17: Amongst these they who worship me with the divine knowledge, and are consistently and absolutely devoted to me, are considered to be best by Me. I am very dear to them and they are dear to me.

BG 7.18: Indeed, Noble are all those who are devoted to me. But those masters of knowledge or wisdom (Jnani), who have a steadfast mind, whose intellect is united in me, and who have made me alone as their supreme goal, I consider them as my very self.

BG 7.19: After following the spiritual path in many births, one who is bestowed with knowledge surrenders unto me, knowing me to be all that is. Such a great person is indeed very exceptional and rare.

BG 7.20: Those whose knowledge has been caught in material desires worship the heavenly gods. Following their own nature, they worship the Devatas, practicing rituals meant to please these godly beings.

BG 7.21: Whatever godly form a devotee seeks to worship with faith, I bless the fruits of such faith in their desired form.

BG 7.22: Gifted with faith, the devotee worships a particular heavenly god and fulfils the objects of desire. But in reality, I alone coordinate these fruits.

BG 7.23: But the fruit gained by these people of limited understanding is perishable. Those who worship the heavenly gods go to the godly abodes, while my devotees come to me.

BG 7.24: The less intelligent believe that I, the Supreme Lord Shree Krishna, was formless earlier and have now form being born in this personality. They do not understand the imperishable glorious nature of my divine form.

BG 7.25: I am not obvious and evident to everyone, being obscured by my divine Yogamaya energy. Hence, those without true knowledge do not know that I am free from birth, unchanging and eternal.

"O Divine, you have a divine form. Only those whose hearts are refined can know you by your grace." (The Ramayana)

BG 7.26: O Arjun, I know the past, the present, and the future, and I also know all living beings; but no one knows me.

"Divine is all-knowing and omniscient. His austerity consists of True knowledge." (Mundakopanishad 1.1.9)
"Divine is beyond the possibility of our logical intelligence." (Kathopanishad 1.2.9)
"Divine cannot be analysed by arguments or reached by words, mind, and intellect." (Ramayan)

BG 7.27: O descendant of Bharat, the dualities of desire and aversion (raga, dvesha) arise from illusion. O conqueror of enemies, all living beings in the material realm are deluded by these from birth.

BG 7.28: But persons, whose sins have been purified and removed by engaging in virtuous activities, become free from the illusion of dualities. Such persons worship me with determination or with virtuous stability.

BG 7.29: Those who take refuge totally (the individual self, and the entire field of karmic action) onto me, endeavouring for liberation from old-age and death, come to know Brahman.

BG 7.30: Those who see me as the governing principle of the adhibhūta (field of the matter) and the adhidaiva (the heavenly gods), and as adhiyajña (the Divine of all sacrificial performances), such enlightened beings are absorbed in absolute consciousness of me even at the time of death.

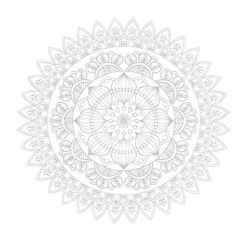

Chapter 8
Eternal Brahman;
Akshara Brahma Yoga

Lord Krishna concluded the seventh chapter by glorifying all-knowing-devotee (Jnani-bhakta) as one who knows and experienced Brahman (Supreme Divine), Adhyatma (science of spirit), Karma (science of action), Adhibhuta and Adhiyajna (the creative and unmanifest nature of the divine).

In this chapter Arjuna asks seven questions of Krishna to understand some of the above terms about Absolute Consciousness.

Lord Krishna explains that the Bhrahman is immortal, eternal, and never-ending Truth. Adhya-Atman is the same as the Brahman behind the individual existence or manifestation. All our actions or Karma are the cause for the birth of all beings. (B.G. 8.3)

Adhibhuta is the entire manifested changeable inert universe. Adhidaiva (creative aspect of divine) is the is the Hiranyagarbha (cosmic golden womb) from which all the organs of all living beings are being created and blessed. Adhiyajna is the Divine principle governing all the Karma or actions of the individual. (B.G. 8.4)

From the 5th verse onward in this chapter, Lord Krishna explains on how to remember the Divine even at the moment of death. The predominant thought-pattern at the time of death determines the place and type of one's next birth. If a person desires for the divine at the moment of death, his rebirth will be favourable for the spiritual path and naturally lead to success in Self-Realisation. The thought pattern at the time of death is determined and governed by one's own predominant thought pattern, Karma and Samaskaras throughout the life. One should try to remember and contemplate about and upon the Divine all the time in order to remember him at the time of death. It may seem very difficult, but by continuous effort, faith and sincere practice (Abhyasa) it is achievable. (B.G. 8.5 to 8)

It is known by Yogis and spiritual seekers that "those who are Saguna-Upasakas will go to Bhrama-Loka. They will attain liberation through blessings of Brahma, the creator himself. This is known as Krama-mukti or freedom from birth cycles.

In the next verses Krishna explains the process of Upasana or Sadhana at the time of death. One should discipline the sense organs (Jnanendriyas) and instruments of action (Karmendriyas). Then by skillful Yoga Sadhana, Prana should be withdrawn from the outward flow and redirected to flow through the Sushumna Nadi to the top of head between the eyebrows. Then the Sadhaka should focus the mind back to the heart, the source or origin of the mind or Chitta. With such a focussed mind, one should meditate upon Omkara or any chosen form of the divine with absolute devotion. One will surely attain Divine realisation, who is omniscient, eternal, the governing principle of all, subtler than the subtlest, sustainer of all, beyond sensory experience, effulgent, and all-knowing. All forms of Tapas or disciplines are to attain oneness with this reality. This is the ultimate goal of Upasana. (B.G. 8.9 to 13)

The Divine is easily realised or attained by sincere meditation and devotion in the Supreme Divine. (B.G. 8.14)

There are two types of goals - Iswara or divine and Samsara or world. No one can be free from the cycle of birth and death by reaching higher lokas (planes of existence) or by acquiring higher bodies. Krishna mentions that even the Brahma, the creator, who has the longest duration of life is not free from the end or death. Everything manifest during the day of Brahma and disappears at the night of Brahma. A day of Brahma is known to be Chatur-Yugas (Satayuga, Tretayuga, Dwaparayuga, and Kaliyuga). So all Lokas or planes of existence are impermanent and finite. Divine is the only eternal and non-changing principle which is beyond the unmanifest and manifest creation or Prakriti. The Divine principle is eternal and is the supreme goal of life. All living beings exist in Him and He is all pervading. Once one attains oneness with that Supreme Consciousness, they attain freedom from the birth cycles of the mortal world (Samsara). (B.G. 8. 15 to 22)

Attainment of Divine Realisation is the highest goal of each life and on this evolutionary journey each life is aspiring towards that ultimate Union or Samadhi. An Upasaka or Sadhaka attains Krama-mukti by going through various birth paths (Sukla-gati) which is primarily governed by the deities of fire, day, bright-fortnight (the waxing moon) and uttarayanam. These seekers go to Brahma-Loka and gain Atma-Jnana or Truth from Brahma himself, and attain liberation. The second type of Upasakas or Path is to follow the rituals of the dark path (Krishna-gati), which is governed by the deities of night, smoke, dark-fortnight and daskhinayanam. Followers of Krishna-Gati return back to the life cycle after enjoying the heavenly fruits of their rituals. (B.G. 8. 23 to 26)

The Sukla-gati or path of light leads one to Divine Realisation and hence one should choose that path alone. To follow that path one should be well established in Upasana and become a Upasaka. Krishna asks Arjuna to be firm and committed to Upasana. (B.G. 8. 27)

Krishna concludes that fruits of Upasana are superior to all other fruits attained through all other means and paths, as it leads the Sadhaka to Supreme-Realisation or Oneness with the Divine.

Upasana will take a seeker to the Guru and Shastra or scriptures. The Upasaka becomes Jnani-bhakta and attains liberation in this life itself.

Eternal Brahman; Akshara Brahma Yoga

BG 8.1-2: Arjun said: O Bhagavan, what is Brahman (Supreme Consciousness), what is adhyātma (the individual consciousness), and what is Karma? What is adhibhuta, and who is Adhidaiva? Who is Adhiyajna in the body and how is He the Adhiyajna? O Krishna, how can You (Supreme Divine) be known at the time of death by those who mastered a steadfast mind (sthita-Prajna)?

BG 8.3: The Divine Krishna said: The Supreme Immortal Being is known as Brahman; one's Individual Self is known as adhyātma. Actions pertaining to the material personality of living beings, and its maturity are known as karma, or fruitive activities (Phala-Karma).

BG 8.4: O best of the living souls (Jivatma), the physical manifestation that is continually changing is known to be adhibhuta; the universal manifested form of Divine, which is presided or governed over the heavenly gods in this creation, is known as adhidaiva; Adhiyajna is the I, who resides in the heart of every living being, who is the Divine of all sacrifices and rituals.

BG 8.5: Those who leave their body while thinking of Me at the moment of death will attain Me. There is certainly no doubt about this.

BG 8.6: Whatever one remembers at the time of leaving the body at the time of death, O son of Kunti, one attains that state. These thoughts will be caused from the whole life and thought pattern that person is involved in.

Story of King Bharata:

BG 8.7: Therefore, always remember Me while do you are doing your duty of taking part in the battle. There is no doubt that "With your mind and intellect merged into Me, you will definitely attain Me".

sumiran ki sudhi yon karo, jyaun gagar panihara
bolat dolat surati men, kahe kabira vichar (Poet Kabir)
"Remember the Divine in all activities just as the woman remembers the
water pot on her head (holding on to it and maintaining the balance),
while she speaks with others and walks on the path."

BG 8.8: With Yoga practice (Yoga-Abhyasa), O Parth, when you continuously engage the mind in remembering Me, the Supreme Divine Consciousness, without deviation, you will certainly attain Me.

BG 8.9-10: The Divine is Omniscient, the one without the beginning or the end, the governing principle of all, subtler than the subtlest, the Sustaining principle of all, He holds an inconceivable divine form; He is brighter than the sun, and beyond all darkness of ignorance. One who at the time of death, with steadfast mind attained by the practice of Yoga, directs the prana (vital life force) between the eyebrows, and steadily remembers the Supreme Consciousness with great devotion, certainly attains Him.

BG 8.11: The Vedas describe Him as Immortal; great ascetics practice the virtue of celibacy and renounce worldly pleasures to attain oneness with Him. Now I shall explain to you the path to that goal of Divine Realisation.

BG 8.12: Closing all the gates of the body (Pratyahara of Cognitive and Locomotive sensory organs) and focussing the mind in the heart region, and then directing the Prana or the vital life force to the crown, one should attain steadfast Yogic concentration (Yoga Dharna).

BG 8.13: One who leaves the body while remembering Me, the Supreme Consciousness, and chanting the mantra Om, will attain the supreme goal of life.

The Vedic scriptures mention that the Divine created sound first at the beginning of creation. With sound he created Akasha or Voidness and continued further. That primodrdial sound is known as Pranava OM. Omkara is the sound manifestation of Supreme Consciousness or Brahman. It represents the vibratory field of the formless aspect of Divine.

BG 8.14: O Parth, for those yogis who always remember Me with total devotion, I am easily attainable to them because of their constant absorption or union in Me.

mām ekam eva śharanam ātmānam sarva-dehinām   (Bhagavatam
11.12.15)
"Devote to Me alone, as the Supreme Consciousness of all living beings."
eka bharoso eka bala ek āsa visvāsa   (Ramayan)
"I have only one practice, one strength, one faith, one refuge, and that is
Shree Ram."
anyāśhrayānām tyāgo 'nanyatā   (Nārad Bhakti Darśhan, Sūtra 10)
"Reject all other refuge, and only refuge in the Divine."

BG 8.15: Having attained in Me, the great souls (Maha-Atma) are free from the cycle of rebirth in this world, which is short-lived and full of suffering and grief. These Souls have attained the highest perfection (Param-Siddhi).

BG 8.16: In all the planes of the material creation, up to the highest abode of Brahma, one will be subject to rebirth, O Arjun. But on attaining My Abode, O son of Kunti, there is no further rebirth.

The Vedic scriptures describe seven lower planes of existence below the earthly plane—tal, atal, vital, sutal, talatal, rasatal, patal. These are known as narak or hell. There are also seven higher planes of existence starting from the earthly plane and above—bhūh, bhuvah, swah, mahah, janah, tapah, satyah. These are known as Swarga or heavenly abodes.

BG 8.17: One day of Brahma (kalp) lasts a thousand cycles of the four age cycles known as ChatuYugas (maha yuga) and his night also extends for the same span of time. The wise who knows this understands the reality about day and night.

BG 8.18: At the beginning of Brahma's day, all living beings originate from the unmanifest source or Prakriti. And at the fall of his night, all living beings again merge into their unmanifest source.

BG 8.19: The multitudes of living beings repeatedly take birth with the beginning of Brahma's day, and are reabsorbed on the arrival of the cosmic night, to manifest again spontaneously at the start of the next cosmic day.

BG 8.20: there is another eternal unmanifest cosmic loka or dimension beyond this manifest and unmanifest creation.

That divine loka or realm does not cease even when all others do.

BG 8.21: That unmanifest loka or plane is the supreme goal, and upon reaching it, one never returns to this mortal world. That is My Supreme Abode.

BG 8.22: The Supreme Divine Consciousness is greater than all that exists. Although He is all-pervading and all living beings are found in Him, He can be known only through devotion.

bhaktyāhamekayā grāhyah śhraddhayātmā priyah satām
(Bhagavatam 11.14.21)

"I am only attained by My devotees who worship Me with faith and love."
milahin na raghupati binu anurāgā, kien joga tapa gyāna birāgā
(Ramayan)
"One may practice ashtanga-yoga, engage in austerities, accumulate knowledge, and develop detachment. Yet, without devotion, one will never attain Supreme Consciousness or oneness with the Divine."

BG 8.23-24: I shall now describe to you the different paths of passing through this world (Samsara), O best of the Bharatas, one of which leads to liberation and the other leads to rebirth. Those who know and attain the Supreme Brahman (creative aspect of the divine), and who leave from this world in Shukla-Paksha or Gati, during the six months of the sun's northern course, the bright fortnight of the moon, and the bright part of the day, attain the supreme goal.

BG 8.25-26: The practitioners of Vedic rituals, who pass away during (the Krishna Paksha or Gati) the six months of the sun's southern course, the dark fortnight of the moon, the time of smoke, the night, attain the heavenly abodes. After enjoying heavenly pleasures, they again return to the earth. These two, bright and dark paths, always exist in this world. The way of light leads to liberation and the way of darkness leads to rebirth.

BG 8.27: Yogis who know the secret of these two paths, O Parth, are never confused. Therefore, at all times remain established in Yoga (union with the Divine).

BG 8.28: The yogis who know this secret gain virtue far beyond the fruits of Vedic rituals, the study of the Vedas, performance of sacrifices, austerities, and charities. Such yogis reach the Supreme Abode of the Divine.

nema dharma āchāra tapa gyāna jagya japa dāna,
bheshaja puni kotinha nahit roga jāhin harijāna. (The Ramayan)

"You may engage in good conduct, righteousness, austerities, sacrifices, ashtanga-yoga, chanting of mantras, and charity. But without devotion to the Divine, the mind's suffering of material consciousness will not cease."

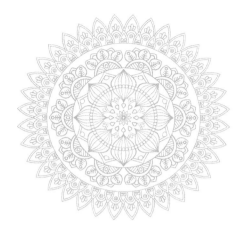

Chapter 9
The Royal Secret;
Raja-vidya or Raja Yoga

The teachings on Upasana or meditation on the absolute divine with the form, qualities and attributions (saguna-upasana) is also not the end goal, but to prepare us for Nirguna-Upasana or attaining oneness with the Absolute Formless Divine free from qualities and attributions. The Saguna Upasana is a means to attain freedom from birth cycles (Krama-mukti) and qualify for absolute liberation of Jivan-Mukti.

Krishna begins the ninth chapter by explaining the saguna and the nirguna forms (jnana and vijnana) of the divine, its glory and required qualifications to experience that absolute cosmic consciousness. Krishna mentions that this is the most sacred wisdom (Raja-Guhya-Vidya) which liberates the knower from the mortal cycle or bondage. It is the easiest and quickest of the paths in bringing fruits of liberation. A Sadhaka should have faith in the Guru, and the teachings for the success in this Yoga.

Further Krisha reveals His true nature to Arjuna. He pervades the whole universe, but is still not related to anything. In reality, there is nothing else existing other than the Absolute Divine. All that is subject to sensory experience appears from and of the Divine Maya. He is eternally and timelessly non-dual (advaita) and free from relativity like the Akasha or space (Keval and Asanga). (B.G. 9. 4 to 6)

The Cosmic Divine is the seed or basis of creation, existence and dissolution of the entire universe (Jagat-Kaaranaam). The cycle of creation dynamically keeps going by the blessings of the Divine. His Prakriti is inseparable from Him. Even though the Divine presence is behind all these dynamic universal phenomena, still He is not involved in any of these as a doer, creator, enjoyer or consumer. The Cosmic Divine is Akarta or non-doer and Abhokta (non-consumer). (B.G. 9. 7 to 10)
Ignorance or Avidya is the key cause of bondage and not knowing the nature of the Divine. Due to ignorance, most living beings see the materials, objects, birth, body, form, etc. as Reality or Divine. This leads to delusion regarding the true nature of the Absolute creative Divine and Individual Jiva or Soul.

This Avidya or ignorance is universal, but most do not even know it or accept it. Here ignorance is believing in material objects, forms and births as REALITY. These people will never even attempt to be free of this Avidya. Not believing in scriptures, these ancient wisdom teachings, and in the established traditions (Paramparai), one may follow another path directed by their senses, desires and attachments it is said.

Also there are noble people who recognise the bondage and avidya and follow the virtuous path to the Divine and seek Him only to be free of the bondage. Krishna mentions that his devotees follow Him in various ways. Some see the Divine or Higher Self in themselves as identical with the Self. Others see Him as different and superior from themselves. While others see Him in everything. His cosmic form is Visvatomukhatvam. (B.G. 9. 13 to 17)

Shree Bhagawan mentions that there are two types of devotees:- those who follow the divine for worldly fruits which are finite in nature (Sakam-Bhaktas) and those who seek the divine path for oneness with the infinite supreme Divine (niskama-bhaktas). Both the paths are fruitful. If we follow the divine for the sake of worldly fruits, we will be blessed with the fruits, but these are limited in nature and hence cannot last for long. A Niskama-bhakta seeks Divine realisation and nothing else, which is eternal, endless and everlasting. Lord Krishna promises that he also takes care of his devotees following the virtuous path for worldly prosperity and wellbeing. (B.G. 9. 18 to 22)

Krishna mentions that it is one's individual choice (Purushartha) to continue and follow the Samasara Marga (path of bondage) or Moksha Marga (path to liberation). When people are following the path of worship and rituals and invoking various aspects of heavenly Gods, then they are invoking the limited qualities of that Infinite Supreme Divine only. All our prayers go to the one ultimate Divine. The amount of water we can fetch from a river depends on the size of the vessel we use, similarly what we receive from the divine is dependent upon our intentions, devotion, faith, and the vidya or knowledge we possess. Many of us miss this divine blessing due to being caught in ignorance. The Divine only blesses us with what we are capable of receiving, as well as willing to receive. So we get what we are seeking for. (B.G. 9. 23 to 25)

A Bhakti or devotion for a Niskama Bhakta is very simple. One can offer anything they like. In Bhakti Marga the attitude, heart and emotion or feeling is most important. Also one should offer every action to the divine purpose mentally (mansika) as part of Bhakti. Such a Bhakta is a Karma Yogi (continuing to fulfil all the duties with no desire to fruits and maintaining equanimity) as well as a Sannyasi (as he has renounced the fruits and attachments). He attains purification and liberation by receiving the scriptural teachings from a Guru. The Divine is available to us all equally, it is down to us to attain or claim Him according to Krishna. (B.G. 9. 26 to 29)

Krishna concludes this chapter by detailing the glories and beauty of Bhakti Marga. Krishna says that "even those who are not qualified for atma-jnana (self-knowledge) because of their past sins, samskaras, weakness, material and extrovert living can attain the Supreme Divine by following the Bhakti Marga. Bhakti is universal and applicable for all. A devotee will never perish.

Krishna advises sadhakas to "keep the mind focused on the Divine, be His devotee, Keep the Divine in mind always, have the Divine as the supreme goal, be His worshiper, surrender to Him. Thus, fixing the mind on Me alone, one will attain Me as the Self". Bhakti is path of love for the divine or meditation on Saguna-Iswara. Krishna also mentions that the Guru is "one who can bless us with self-knowledge (atma-jnana) alone can lead one directly to liberation."

The Royal Secret;
Raja-vidya or Raja Yoga

BG 9.1: Shree Bhagavan said: O Arjun, because you are not envious of Me, I shall now disclose to you this very confidential knowledge and wisdom (guhya-vidya), upon knowing which you will be released from the miseries of material existence.

BG 9.2: This knowledge is the Supreme of all sciences and the most profound of all secrets. It refines (Pavitram) those who hear it. It is individually attainable, in accordance with dharma, easy to practice, and everlasting in effect. "Bhakti destroys the three poisons—pāp (sins), bīja (the seed of sins), avidyā (the ignorance in the heart)."

BG 9.3: O defeater of enemies, people who have no faith in this dharma (ashardhanah) are unable to attain Me. They repeatedly come back to this world (samasara) in the cycle of birth and death.

BG 9.4: My unmanifest formless Cosmic Consciousness pervades the entire cosmic manifestation (Jagat). All living beings (Jivas) reside in Me, but I do not inhabit in them.

eko devah sarvabhūteshu gūdhah sarvavyāpī (Śhwetāśhvatar
Upanishad 6.11)
"There is one Divine; He is contained in everyone's heart; He is also universally in this world."

īśhāvāsyam idam sarvam yat kiñcha jagatyām jagat (Īśhopanishad 1)
"God is everywhere and all-pervading in this universe."

purusha evedam sarvam, yad bhūtam yachcha bhavyam (Purush
Sūktam)
"God pervades everything that has existed and all that will exist."

BG 9.5: And yet, the living beings do not abide in Me. Behold the mystery of My divine energy! Although I am the Creator and Preserver of all living beings, I am not influenced by the living beings (Jiva Shakti) or by the material nature (Maya Shakti).

BG 9.6: Like the mighty wind blowing everywhere remains always in the Akasha or voidness, likewise all living beings rest always in Me. This verse means "all living beings rest in Cosmic Consciousness."

BG 9.7-8: At the end of one Kalp, all living beings merge into My primordial material energy (Manifested Para-Prakriti). At the beginning of the next creation, O son of Kunti, I manifest them again. Governing over My material energy, I create these countless forms again and again, in accordance with the force of their natures.

BG 9.9: O Dhananjaya (master or victor of wealth), I am not bound to any of these actions. I remain like a neutral observer (Drashta-Bhava), ever detached from these actions.

"The material energy is lifeless by itself. But when it receives creativeness from the Divine, it begins to act as if it were conscious or living." (The Ramayana)

BG 9.10: Operating under My guidance, this material energy brings into being all living and non-living forms, O son of Kunti. For this purpose, the material world undergoes the changes (creation, continuation, and dissolution).

BG 9.11: When I appear in My personal form deluded individuals are unable to acknowledge Me. They do not know the divinity of My personality, as the Supreme Lord (Iswara) of all beings.

"I had the vision of God as a boy who is never overpowered, and who appeared in a family of cowherds." (Rig Veda 1.22.164 sūkta 31)

"The Lord, wearing a garland of forest flowers, plays His flute, enchantingly forming the mauna mudrā with His hands." (Gopāl Tāpani Upanishad 1.13)

"The deepest Vidya to know is that God accepts a human-like form." (Bhagavatam 7.15.75)
"At that time, the Supreme Lord, who occupies all abundance, appeared in a human-like form." (Bhagavatam 9.23.20)

Brahma prays to Shree Krishna, "I worship Lord Krishna whose form is eternal, all-knowing, and blissful. He is without beginning and end and is the cause of all causes." (Brahma Samhitā 5.1)

BG 9.12: Confused by the material energy, such persons embrace and follow demoniac and atheistic views. In that deluded state, their hopes for welfare are in vain, their fruitive actions are wasted, and their culture of knowledge is confused.

BG 9.13: But the great souls (Maha-Atmana), who take refuge in My Divine Consciousness, O Parth, know Me, Lord Krishna, as the source of all creation. They participate in My devotion with their minds fixed absolutely on Me.

BG 9.14: Always singing My divine glories (Kirtan), striving with great determination(Dradha-Vratta), and humbly bowing down before Me (Namastasya), they constantly worship Me in devotional love (Bhakti-prema).

Kīrtan is one of the most powerful means of Bhakti Sadhana. It involves the three-fold devotion of Shravana (hearing), kirtan (singing), and smarana (remembering).

"The best Bhakti Sadhana Path in the age of Satya Yuga was simple meditation upon God. In the age of Treta Yuga, it was the performance of sacrifices for the gratification of God. In the age of Dwapar Yuga, worship of the deities was the recommended process. In the present age of Kali Yuga, it is kirtan alone." (Bhagavatam 12.3.52)

BG 9.15: Bhaktas follow or worship Me in many forms. Some worship me by engaging in the Jnana-yajna of cultivating knowledge. Others see Me as identical with their own self which is non-different from them, while others see Me as separate from them. While others worship Me in the infinite manifestations of My cosmic form.

BG 9.16-17: I am the Vedic ritual, I am the sacrifice, and I am the offerings offered to the ancestors. I am the medicinal herb, and I am the Vedic mantra. I am the purified ghee, I am the fire and the act of offering. Of this universe, I am the Father (Pita); I am also the Mother (Mata), the Sustainer (Dhata), and the Grandsire. I am the purifier, the goal of knowledge, the sacred syllable Om. I am the Rig Veda, Sama Veda, and the Yajur Veda.

BG 9.18: I am the Supreme Goal of all living beings (Jivas), and I am also their Sustainer, Master (Prabhu), Witness (Sakshi), Dwelling (Nivasa), Shelter (Sharanam), and Friend (Mitra). I am the Origin, End, and Resting Place of creation (Sthanam); I am the Storehouse (Nidhanam) and Eternal Seed (Bijam).

BG 9.19: I am the light and heat of the sun, and I withhold, as well as send forth rain. I am immortality (amritam) as well as death personified (Mrityu), O Arjun. I am the soul as well as the matter.

Shree Krishna says to Brahma: "I am all that exists, or all that is to exist and all that is to be dissolved and that has been dissolved . Prior to creation, I alone existed. Now that creation has come about, whatever is in the form of the manifested world is my very self. After dissolution, I alone will exist. There is nothing apart from Me." (Bhagavatam 2.9.32)

BG 9.20: Those who are motivated towards the fruitive activity described in the Vedas worship Me through ritualistic sacrifices (karma-kanda). Being purified from sin (paap) by drinking the Soma juice, which is the remnant of the Yajnas, they seek to go to heaven (swarga-lokah). By virtue of their pious deeds, they go to the abode of Indra (Indra-lokah), the king of heaven, and enjoy the pleasures of the heavenly gods (Deva-bhogah).

BG 9.21: When they have enjoyed the cosmic pleasures of heaven, once the stock of their fruits has been exhausted, they return to the earthly plane (Bhuloka). Thus, those who follow the Vedic rituals, desiring objects of enjoyment, repeatedly come and go in this world (Samsarika Jivan-Mrityu Chakra).
"Dwellers of heaven relish the heavenly delights until their accumulated Karmic assets have been exhausted. Then they are reluctantly forced to fall back to the lower abodes by the passage of time." (Bhagavatam 11.10.26)

"The attainment of heaven is temporary, and is followed by miseries." (Ramayan)
"The human form is especially rare. Even the heavenly deities pray to attain it." (Nārad Purān)

BG 9.22: There are people (Janah) who always think of Me and engage in absolute devotion to Me. To them, whose minds are always absorbed in Me (Nitya-Abhiyuktam), I provide what they lack and preserve what they already hold.

BG 9.23: O son of Kunti, even those devotees who devotedly worship other deities also worship Me. But they do so with limited knowledge.

"When we water the root of a tree, its trunk, branches, twigs, leaves, and flowers all are nourished. When we eat food, it nourishes the life energy currents (Prana-Vayus) and the senses automatically. In the same way, by worshipping the Supreme Lord, all other aspects and forms of gods and goddesses are also being worshipped." (Bhagavatam 4.31.14)

BG 9.24: I am the enjoyer and the only Master and Lord (Prabhu or Iswara) of all sacrifices. But those who fail to comprehend My divine nature are subject to be reborn.

BG 9.25: Worshippers of the heavenly gods take birth amongst the heavenly gods, worshippers of the ancestors go to the ancestors, worshippers of ghosts take birth amongst such beings, and My devotees come to Me alone.

BG 9.26: If one offers a leaf, a flower, a fruit, or even the water to Me with devotion I delightfully accept that article offered with love by My devotee in pure consciousness.

"If you offer God with sincere love just a Tulsī leaf, and as much water as you can hold in your palm, He will offer Himself to you in return because He is endeared by love." (Hari-Bhakta-Vilas)

BG 9.27: Whatever you do, whatever you eat, whatever you offer to the sacred fire (Yajna-agni), whatever gift you present, and whatever austerities (Tapsya) you perform, O son of Kunti, do them as an offering to Me.

"Devotion means offering your every action to God, and feeling such intense union with the Divine that you cannot bare to lose him for even a moment" (Nārad Bhakti Darśhan, Sūtra 19)

"Wherever I walk, I feel I am performing the pilgrim-circling of the Lord's temple; whatever I do, I see it as service to God. When I go to sleep, I meditate on the sentiment that I am offering obeisance to God. In this way, I remain ever united with Him." (Saint Kabir)

BG 9.28: By dedicating all your deeds or actions (Karmas) to Me, you will be freed from the bondage of good and bad fruits. With your mind committed to Me through renunciation, you will be liberated and will certainly reach Me.

BG 9.29: I am equally with all living beings; I am neither unfriendly nor partial to anyone. But the devotees who worship Me with love reside in Me and I reside in them.

The rainwater falls equally upon the earth. Yet, the drop that falls on the cornfields gets converted into grain; the drop that falls on the desert bush gets converted into a thorn; the drop that falls in the gutter becomes dirty water; and the drop that falls in the oyster becomes a pearl. There is no partiality on the part of the rain, since it is equitable in bestowing its grace upon the land. The raindrops cannot be held responsible for this variation in results, which are a consequence of the nature of the recipient. Similarly, God states here that He is equally disposed toward all living beings, and yet, those who do not love Him are bereft of the benefits of His grace because their hearts are unsuitable vessels for receiving it.

BG 9.30: Even if the evilest sinners worship Me with total devotion (ananya-bhakti), they are to be considered righteous, for they have made the proper resolve.

BG 9.31: Swiftly they become virtuous and attain everlasting peace (shasvata-shanti). O son of Kunti, declare it confidently that no devotee of Mine is ever lost.

BG 9.32: All those who take refuge in Me, whatever their birth, race, sex, or caste, even those whom society scorns, will attain the supreme destination.

The Padam Purana states that God is not concerned with the time or place where we perform devotion. He only appreciates the love in our heart. All souls are the children of God, and He is willing to accept everyone with open arms, provided they come to Him with genuine love." (Padma Puran)

BG 9.33: What then to speak about kings and sages with admirable deeds? Therefore, having come to this momentary and joyless world, engage in devotion unto Me.

BG 9.34: Always contemplate Me, be dedicated to Me, adore Me, and offer respect to Me. Having dedicated your mind and body to Me, you will certainly come to Me.

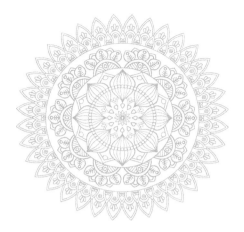

Chapter 10
Divine Glories of Bhagavan;
Vibhuti Yoga

In the last chapter, Krishna explained that the Divine is the material cause of the universe. Like the action follows the reaction, or the effect is not different from the material cause, similarly the universe is indifferent from the Divine. Hence the whole universe is the cosmic manifestation of Divine Consciousness. All the glories of our dynamic and cosmic manifestation belong to the Divine itself.

Vibhuti means the siddhis, or qualities, while yoga is the path, practice and end goal to manifest union with divine consciousness. In this chapter Krishna details Vibhuti Yoga or absolute qualities and glories of the divine. He mentions that even the great sages (Sadhus) cannot speak about the glories of the supreme divine or the Prabhu, as they are limited beings in the body. This is the rarest of knowledge that has been ever given. One who attains this knowledge, surely attains liberation from the ocean of Samaskara. (B.G. 10.1 to 3) Krishna mentions that the entire gross universe of material manifestation and the subtle universe of thoughts originate from Him. The seven great sages (Sapta-Rishis), four sages, and the Manus are all born of the mind of the Divine Lord. One who knows and realises this, attains self-knowledge (Atma-Jnana) surely. (B.G. 10.4 to 7)

The great devotees (Virata-Bhakta) accept everything in their life as a divine blessing of the Lord (Prabhu) because the Divine is the source of all and everything. They continually think about the Divine, speak about the Divine, hear about the Divine. They spend every moment of their lives working to experience oneness with the Divine. (B.G. 10.8 to 9)

Still they are Saguna-Bhaktas. Krishna says that "He takes the responsibility to enlighten them. Out of His love and compassion for the Bhaktas, the Divine Lord lights up the lamps of wisdom, by remaining in their heart. Here according to the Upanishads it is believed that the Lord blesses His Bhaktas with the Guru and ideal conditions for the Jnana and Nirguna-Bhakti (absolute knowledge and highest love for divine). (B.G. 10.10 to 11)

Arjuna requests Krishna to bless him with details of His Cosmic glories, which can help him in his Upasana or worship and meditation. (B.G. 10.12 to 18)

From the 19th verse onward in this chapter, Krishna describes His Glories as the Bhagavan or Supreme Lord. He mentions that these are just a few of the important ones, not the beginning or the end of His glories. No one can ever detail all the glories of the Divine Lord. (B.G. 10.19 & 40)

Krishna begins with details of the absolute Self and mentions that "the best, the closest and the most evident expression of the Divine is the 'self', 'I', the consciousness. Krishna concludes this by mentioning that "He is the true and primordial existence in all beings, because He is the material seed cause (bijam) of all. All that exists, and their qualities and glories are the expressions of only a ray of glories of the Divine.

Ultimate reality is that "the entire universe is in the Divine and occupies a part of Him as if it were." In reality the universe is part of the Divine as his manifested matter or nature.

Divine Glories of Bhagavan; Vibhuti Yoga

BG 10.1: The Shree Bhagavan said: O mighty armed one, listen to my divine teachings. I shall reveal them to you as you are my beloved friend and I Desire your welfare.

BG 10.2: Neither heavenly gods (Devas) nor the great sages (Maha-Rishis) know my origin. I am the source from which the gods and great Rishis originate from.

"Who in the world can know clearly? Who can declare from where this universe was born? Who can state where this creation has come from? The Devatas came to existence after creation. Therefore, who knows from where the universe arose?" (The Rig Veda)

"God cannot be known by the heavenly Devatas, as he existed before them." (Ishopanishad 4)[v2]

BG 10.3: Those who know me as one who never being born (Ajanma) and beginningless (Anadi), and as the Supreme Divine of the universe (Maha-ishwaraha), those are free from illusion and emancipated from all evils among the mortal beings.

"The Supreme Divine is the Regulator of all regulators; he is the God of all gods. He is the Beloved of all beloveds; he is the Ruler of the world, and beyond the material energy." (the Śhwetāśhvatar Upanishad)

BG 10.4-5: All the varieties in the qualities of moods, thoughts and feelings amongst humans arise from my powers only. Krishna here mentions the following qualities:

Buddhi - Intellect or the ability to analyse things with the appropriate perspective.

Jnanam - knowledge or the ability to discriminate eternal from mortal.

A-sammoham - ability to be free from the confusion or hypnosis from mundane maya.

Kshama - Forgiveness or the ability to forgive.

Satyam - Truth or the ability to follow truth and honesty at all levels.

Dam - Sensory Withdrawal or ability to restrain senses from the object of senses.

Sham - Discipline of mind.

Sukham - Pleasant Being or the state of being at ease, experiencing joy and delight.

Duhkham - The feeling or emotion of pain, sorrow and affliction.

Bhavah - The knowing that 'I exist".

A-bhavah -The realisation or knowing of death.

Bhaya - The fear of advancing troubles.

Abhaya - Fearlessness or the freedom from fear.

Ahimsha - Non-violence or ability to abstain from any form of harm.

Samata - Equanimity in pain and pleasure.

Tushti - Contentment or feeling content with the fruits of one's karma.

Tapa - Disciplined Practice or voluntary austerities for spiritual evolution.

Dan - Charity or giving what we can to the needy or the one who is worthy.

Yash - Fame due to virtuous qualities.

Ayaah - Disgrace for non-virtuous or evil qualities.

BG 10.6: The four great Saints, the seven great Sages (Sapta-Rishi), and the fourteen Manus, are all born from My mind. All the people in the world have descended from Them.

Brahma was born from the Hiranyagarbh, the cosmic energy of Vishnu. Brahma created the four great saints (Sanak, Sanandan, Sanat, Sanatan) also known as the four Kumaras. In our universe, the four Kumaras are the oldest and first creation of Brahma. These were born from the power of the mind of Brahma and hence have no mother. They were eternally liberated souls and masters of Yoga and Atma-Jnana, these Kumaras were empowered to help others attain liberation through spiritual sadhana. It is believed that they are still there helping the Bhaktas and Seekers of the Divine.

After the four Kumaras, Brahma created Sapta-Rishis or seven sages:- Mareech, Angira, Atri, Pulastya, Pulaha, Kratu, and Vasishtha. These great rishis were empowered with the task of procreation of the human population.

Then the fourteen Manus were created to administer the human kind and establish Vedic or Sanatan Dharma for peace and prosperity on earth. These were Svayambhuva, Swarochisha, Uttam, Tamas, Raivat, Chakshusha, Vaivasvat, Savarni, Dakshasavarni, Brahmasavarni, Dharmasavarni, Rudra-putra, Rochya, and Bhautyaka.

We are presently in the era of the seventh Manu, who is called Vaivasvat Manu. This era is thus called Vaivasvat Manvantar. In the present kalp (day of Brahma), there will be seven more Manus.

BG 10.7: Those who know My True glories (Vibhuti) and divine powers attain union (Yoga) with me through steadfast bhakti yoga. There is no doubt about this.

The word vibhuti here refers to the great shaktis (powers) and siddhis (miracles) and glories of the Divine manifesting in this universe. The word Yoga refers to the Divine's connection with these glorious and miraculous powers.

BG 10.8: I am the origin of all creation (sarvasya). "I am the Supreme Ultimate Truth and the cause of all causes." Everything advances from me. The wise who know this perfectly worship me with great faith and devotion.

"Infinite universes—each have Shankar, Brahma, and Vishnu—manifest from the openings of Maha Vishnu's body when he breathes in, and

again dissolve into him when he breathes out. I worship Shree Krishna of whom Maha Vishnu is an expansion." (Brahma Samhitā 5.48)

"I bring glory and prosperity to people I love; I make them men or women; I make them wise sages; I create a soul empowered for the seat of Brahma." (The Rig Veda 10.125.5)

BG 10.9: With their minds (Chitta) fixed on Me and their life (Prana) surrendered to Me, My devotees (Bhakta) remain ever satisfied (Tu-shyanti) in Me. They spring great gratification and bliss in sharing and helping one another in this enlightening glory (Satsanga) about Me.

This verse gives us another Sadhana in day-to-day life. The Bhaktas or devotees love their Lord and praise His glories in their speech. They engage in speaking, listening, singing and acting out the names, forms, virtues, pastimes, abodes, and devotees of the Supreme Divine (Maha-Prabhu). They engage in kirtan (singing and chanting) and shravana (hearing) regarding the glories of God, they relish his sweetness for themselves and share it with others as well. They contribute to eachother's progress by enlightening others about the divine knowledge of God (bodhayanti). Speaking and singing about the glories of God gives the devotees great satisfaction (tushyanti), and delight (ramanti). In this way, they worship him through the processes of remembering, hearing, and chanting. This is the threefold bhakti comprising of shravana, kirtan, and samarana.

BG 10.10: I bless the divine knowledge by which they can attain Me to those who keep their minds united with Me.

Our thoughts, understanding, and wisdom are limited to the material realm while the Divine and his divine realm are entirely beyond the scope of our worldly intellect. The only way to know the divine, is by transcending the worldly limited perception by grace of the Divine Vision.

"Those who think they can know God with their intellects have no understanding of God. Only those who know that he is beyond the scope of their comprehension truly know him." (Kenopanishad 2.3)

"One can never realise God by self-effort based upon the worldly intellect." (The Brihadaranyak Upanishad 3.9.26)

"Lord Ram is beyond the scope of our intellect, mind, and words." (The Ramayan)

"Without bathing oneself in the nectar emanating from the lotus feet of God, no one can know him." (The Yajur Veda)

BG 10.11: Out of compassion (anukampa) for them, I, who dwell within their hearts, destroy the darkness born of ignorance (Ajnana), with the luminous lamp of knowledge (Jnana-Deep).

BG 10.12-13: Arjun said: You are the Supreme Divine Self (Parmatman), the Supreme Abode (Dhama), the Supreme Purifier (Pavitram), the Eternal God (Shasavtam), the Primal Being (adi-deva), the Unborn (Ajanma), and the Greatest. The great sages, like Narad, Asit, Deval, and Vyas, declared this, and now You, Yourself are declaring it to me.

Sage Narad: "Shree Krishna is the creator of all the worlds and the knower of all spirits. He is the Lord of the heavenly gods, who administer the universe."

Sage Markandeya states: "Lord Krishna is the goal of all religious sacrifices (Yajna-Karma) and the essence of austerities. He is the present, past, and future (Vartaman, Bhuta, Bhavisya) of everything."

Sage Bhrigu says: "He is the God of gods and the first original form of Lord Vishnu."

Sage Ved Vyas states: "O Lord Krishna, You are the Lord of the Vasus. You have conferred power on Indra and the other celestial gods."

Sage Angira says: "Lord Krishna is the creator of all beings. All the three worlds exist in his belly. He is the Supreme Personality (Parmatman) of Godhead."

Sage Asit and Deval declare: "Shree Krishna is the creator of Brahma, who is the creator of the three worlds." (Mahabharat Vana Parva 12.50)

BG 10.14: O Krishna, I absolutely acknowledge everything you have stated to me as the Truth. O Lord, neither gods nor the demons can understand your true personality.

"Bhagavan is he who possesses these six abundances to the infinite extent—strength, knowledge, beauty, fame, opulence, and renunciation." (Devi Bhagavad Purana)

BG 10.15: Indeed, you alone know yourself by your inconceivable energy, O Supreme Being, the Creator and Lord of all beings, the God of gods, and the Lord of the universe!

In this verse Arjuna describes the following qualities of Lord Krishna:

Bhuta-bhavana – The Creator of all beings
Bhutesh – the Supreme Master of all beings.
Jagat-pate – the Absolute Master of creation.
Deva-deva – the God of all the heavenly gods.

BG 10.16-17: Please reveal your divine glories to me, by which you pervade all the worlds and reside in them. O Supreme Master of Yoga (Yogeshwar), how may I think of you and know you? And what forms may I envision of you while meditating, O Supreme Divine Being?

BG 10.18: Disclose your divine glories and manifestations to me again, O Janardan. I can never tire of hearing your nectar (Amritam).

"Those who are devoted to Lord Krishna never tire of hearing narratives of his divine amusements. The nectar of these pastimes is such that the more it is appreciated the more it increases." (Srimad Bhagavatam, 1.1.19)

BG 10.19: The Shree Bhagavan spoke: I shall now briefly describe my divine glories to you, O best of the Kurus, there is no beginning or the end to their detail.

"Divine is limitless and manifests in infinite forms in the universe. Although he governs the universe, he is yet the non-doer." (Shwetashvatar Upanishad 1.9)
"Divine is limitless, and the pastimes (Leelas) he enacts in his infinite Avatars are also unlimited." (The Ramayana)

BG 10.20: O Arjun, I am seated in the heart of all living beings. I am the beginning (Adi), middle (Madhyam), and end (antah) of all beings (sarva-bhuta).

"God is the atma of the atma (Soul of the soul) of all living beings." (Srimad Bhagavatam)

"Lord Krishna is the Supreme Soul of all living beings in the universe. For the benefit of humankind, he has appeared in a human form by his

Yogmaya ." (Bhagavatam 10.14.55)

"All living beings have emanated from the Divine; God is He within whom all living beings are situated; God is He into whom all living beings shall unite." (Taittiriya Upanishad 3.1.1)

BG 10.21: Amongst the twelve sons of Aditi I am Vishnu; amongst luminous (Jyoti) objects I am the sun. Know me to be Marichi amongst the Maruts, and the moon amongst the stars (nakshatram) in the night sky.

BG 10.22: Among the Vedas, I am the Sama Veda, and Indra amongst the heavenly gods. I am the mind amongst the senses; amongst the living beings I am consciousness (chetana).

BG 10.23: I am the Shakar amongst the Rudras; I am Kuber amongst the semi-demons. I am Agni amongst the Vasus and Meru amongst the mountains.

The Rudras are the eleven forms of Lord Shiva—Hara, Bahurupa, Tryambaka, Aparajita, Vrisakapi, Shankar, Kapardi, Raivata, Mrigavyadha, Sarva, Kapali.

Yakshas (semi-divine demons) are beings who are very fond of acquiring wealth and hoarding it. Kuber is the god of wealth and the treasurer of the celestial gods.

There are eight Vasus—land, water, fire, air, space, sun, moon, and stars. They constitute the primary structure of the universe. Amongst these, agni (fire) gives warmness and energy to the rest of the elements.

Meru is a mountain in the heavenly abodes famed for its rich natural resources. It is believed to be the axis around which many heavenly bodies rotate.

BG 10.24: O Arjun, I am Brihaspati amongst priests; I am Kartikeya amongst warrior chiefs; and I am the ocean amongst reservoirs of water.

BG 10.25: Amongst the great seers I am Bhrigu and I am the transcendental Om amongst sounds. Know me to be the repetition of the Sacred Term amongst the Chants; I am the Himalayas amongst immovables.

BG 10.26: I am the peepal (a sacred fig tree) amongst trees; I am Narada among the heavenly sages. I am Chitrath amongst the Gandharvas and the sage Kapila amongst the Siddhas.

BG 10.27: Know me to be Ucchaihshrava amongst horses created from the churning of the ocean of nectar. I am Airavata amongst all mighty elephants, and the king amongst humans.

BG 10.28: I am the Vajra (thunderbolt) amongst weapons and Kamadhenu amongst the cows. I am Kaamdev, the god of love, amongst all causes for procreation; I am Vasuki amongst serpents.

BG 10.29: I am Ananta amongst the snakes; I am Varuna amongst aquatics. Amongst the departed ancestors I am Aryama; I am Yamraj, the lord of death amongst law dispensers.

BG 10.30: I am Prahlad amongst the demons; I am time amongst all that controls. Know me to be the lion amongst animals, and Garuda amongst the birds.

BG 10.31: I am the wind amongst purifiers, and amongst warriors and masters of weapons I am Lord Ram. I am the crocodile of water creatures, and I am the Ganga amongst the flowing rivers.

BG 10.32: O Arjun, I am the Creator (adi), Maintainer (madhya), and Annihilator (anta) of all Sarga (space, air, fire, water, and earth, are known as sarga.) or creation. Amongst sciences (Vijnana) I am the science of spirituality (Adhyatma-Vijnana), and in debates I am the logical conclusion.

BG 10.33: I am the beginning "Akaar" amongst all letters; I am the dual word in grammatical compounds. I am the endless Time, and amongst creators I am Brahma.

Dvandwa Samas is a combination of two words where both words still keep their original meaning within the collective meaning, eg. Atmajnana (Atma+Jnana), Yogeshwar (Yoga+Iswara) etc.

BG 10.34: I am the unavoidable Death (Mrityuh), and I am the origin (Udbhavah) of those things that are yet to manifest. I am the Kirti-fame, shri-prosperity, vaak-fine speech, smriti-memory, medha- intelligence, dhriti-courage and Kshama-forgiveness amongst feminine qualities.

BG 10.35: Know me to be the Brihastama amongst the hymns in the Sāma Veda; I am the Gayatri amongst the poetic meters. Of the twelve months of the Hindu calendar I am Margsheersh, and of seasons I am spring, which brings forth flowers.

BG 10.36: I am the gambling of the gamblers and the splendour (Teja) of the splendid (Tejasvi). I am the victory of the victorious, the resolve of the resolute, and the virtue (sattva) of the virtuous (Sattvam).

BG 10.37: Amongst the descendants of Vrishni, I am Krishna, and I am Arjuna amongst the Pandavas. Know me to be Ved Vyas amongst the sages, and Shukracharya amongst the great thinkers (Kavi).

BG 10.38: I am merely punishment amongst means of preventing injustice and chaos, and right conduct and order (Niti) amongst those who seek success. I am silence amongst the secrets, and the wisdom of the wise.

BG 10.39: I am the breeding seed of all living beings, O Arjun. Without me, no organism moving or non-moving can exist.

There four ways living beings are born:

Andaj - born from eggs, such as birds, snakes, and lizards
Jarayuj - born from the womb, such as humans, cows, dogs, and cats
Swedaj - born from sweat, such as lice, ticks, etc
Udbhij - sprouting from the earth, such as trees, creepers, grass, and corn.

BG 10.40: There is no end to my divine manifestations, O conqueror of enemies. What I have declared to you is a mere taster of my endless glories.

BG 10.41: All that you see as beautiful, glorious, or powerful, know it to have originated from Me but as a spark of my splendour.

BG 10.42: O Arjun, What need is there for all this detailed knowledge? Know that by one fraction of my existence, I pervade and support this entire creation.

"This temporary world made from the material energy is merely a part of the Supreme Divine Self. The other three parts are his eternal abodes that are beyond the phenomenon of life and death."
(Purush Suktam Mantra 3)

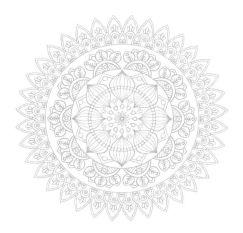

Chapter 11
The Vision of Cosmic Form;
Vishwarupa Darshana Yoga

Krishna has mentioned that the entire universe is material manifestation of Divine Consciousness and revealed His glories. The whole universe belongs to the divine alone and He is all pervading.

This chapter begins with Arjuna summarising the teachings of Krishna so far (the nature of Jiva - Individual self and the nature of Bhagavan - the Supreme Self). Even though Arjuna has received the teachings from Krishna Himself, due to his own limited abilities and mind he is still struggling to comprehend the Universal or Cosmic Form of the Bhagavan or lord. He prays to Krishna to bless him with the vision of universal form of the Supreme Divine. (B.G. 11. 1 to 4)

Here Lord Krishna agrees to bless Arjuna with the divine vision of His Universal Form (Viswa-Rupa). Krishna mentions that, "one cannot see the divine from human ordinary eyes and hence grants Arjuna with the divine eyes to fulfil the purpose. Just remember that the universal form of the divine is not a special form, but rather "it is the divine himself that is the universe." This Viswa-Rupa is available eternally for all at all times and Divine does not need to reveal it to us. We just don't experience IT due to our limited perception. Yoga provides us all the Kriyas and Prakriyas to refine our mind and enhance our ordinary perception ability into divine perception or realisation. The Divine is there in each particle, from each drop of water to each blade of grass and in each living being, tree, as well as all materials. (B.G. 11. 5 to 8)

From verse 9 Sanjay describes the Universal Form of the Divine. He says that "we can picture the divine as a special person with the brilliance of the thousand suns together."

Further from verse 15 Arjuna details the Universal Form and appreciates the Divine Form of Lord Krishna. Arjuna mentions that he see all beings in the cosmic body of the Bhagavan or Lord. The sun and the moon seem to like Krishna's eyes. He sees the hands, feet, legs etc. of the people as of the Lord Himself. He sees Krishna's body with thousands of hands, legs, and other limbs, appearing to be without origin, middle or end. (B.G. 11. 15 to 22)

Further Arjuna sees the mouth of Lord Krishna, which seems to represent the Kala or Death. With the blazing fire and sharp expanded teeth, the vision of the Lord's mouth brings terror in all including Arjuna. Arjuna sees the entire universe being burned by the Kala or fire of death. He sees many entering his mouth, many already in his mouth and many others approaching to be crushed between his teeth. This confuses Arjuna and he begins to doubt if Lord Krishna is a loving creator or a terrifying destroyer. Here it seems that Arjuna is only able to see parts of divine and not the whole (B.G. 11. 23 to 31)

Krishna clarifies here that both the creative and fierce aspects are only Himself manifesting as the Time or Kala principle of birth and death. When it is the time for living beings to die, the Supreme Lord finds the instrument to make this happen. Krishna mentions Arjuna as the instrument of death for many at the battlefield. Arjuna understands now that Krishna, The Cosmic Supreme Divine, is the creator, regulator, manager and dissolution aspects and surrenders totally to His Will and Glory. Now Arjuna realises and appreciates the Wholeness of Krishna as the basis of creation, maintenance and dissolution. Arjuna mentions that other forms of the Divine, everything else is insignificant in context with the Supreme Consciousness. He totally surrenders to Krishna and becomes his devotee or Bhakta and seeks for forgiveness for all his mistakes, faults and actions. (B.G. 11. 32 to 45)

Arjun was blessed to have this divine vision of Supreme Lord, but still somehow struggled to accept the wholeness of Krishna as the dissolution aspect seems to be too terrifying. Arjuna requests Krishna to withdraw His form. (B.G. 11.46)

In the last part of this chapter Krishna withdraws His Universal Form and also takes Arjun's divine eyes (divya-drashti) away to bring him back to human consciousness. Krishna mentions that Bhakti is one of the highest paths to attain this cosmic wisdom. Arjuna was able to receive this experience only because of his sincere devotion. Bhakti helps one in purifying the mind, and enables one to attain realisation of this universal form of the divine and know the absolute true nature of the Lord and become one with the Divine. (B.G. 11. 47 to 55)

Krishna recommends that we all should "Fulfil our Karma for the divine purpose; Practice Devotion to the divine; seek the divine as the ultimate goal; be detached from worldly desires and objects (Vairajna); be free from any form of hate and harm towards all. Such a Sadhaka certainly reaches the Divine."

The Vision of Cosmic Form; Vishwarupa Darshana Yoga

BG 11.1: Arjuna said: Listening to the absolutely confidential spiritual knowledge, which has been revealed to me by you out of compassion, my illusion is now dispelled.

BG 11.2: After hearing it all from You, now I know the truth about the manifestation and vanishing of all living beings, O lotus-eyed one, and also about your eternal magnificence.

BG 11.3: O Supreme Lord, you are absolutely the Supreme Divine exactly as you have revealed yourself to be. Now I wish for the vision of your Divine Cosmic Form (Divya-Vishwa-Rupa), O greatest of the Self.

BG 11.4: O Yogeshwar, I have expressed my wish. If you consider me worthy (Adhikari) of it, then by your grace, please bless me with your Cosmic Form to me, and show me your Yoga-ishwara (Master of Yoga).

BG 11.5: The Supreme Lord said: Witness, O Parth, my hundreds and thousands of wonderful forms (Divya-Rupa) of various shapes, sizes, and colours.

BG 11.6: Witness Me, O offspring of the Bharatas, the (twelve) sons of Aditi, the (eight) Vasus, the (eleven) Rudras, the (twin) Ashwini Kumars, as well as the (forty-nine) Maruts and many more wonders never revealed before.

BG 11.7: Witness now, Arjun, the entire universe (Jagat), with everything moving (Chara) and non-moving (Achara), compiled together in my universal form. Whatever else you wish to witness, observe it all within this universal form.

BG 11.8: But you cannot witness my cosmic form with these human eyes of yours. Therefore, I bless you with divine vision. Witness my magnificent affluence!

BG 11.9: Sanjay said: O King, having spoken thus, the Supreme Master of Yoga (Yogeshwar), Shree Krishna, revealed his divine and magnificent form to Arjun.

BG 11.10-11: In that cosmic divine form (Viswa-Rupa), Arjun is seeing infinite faces and eyes, ornamented with many cosmic ornaments and exercising many kinds of divine weapons. He wore many garlands on his body and was smoothed with many sweet-smelling heavenly fragrances. He revealed himself as the magnificent and infinite Lord whose face is everywhere.

BG 11.12: that absolute magnificent form has the illumination of thousands of suns with unmatched splendour.

BG 11.13: There Arjun witnessed the wholeness of the entire universe founded in one place, in that form of the God of gods.

BG 11.14: Then, Arjun, full of astonishment and with hair standing on end, addressed the Lord with bowed head and folded hands.

"Being bemused, sweating, horrified, the voice choking, trembling, complexion becoming ashen, shedding tears, and fainting—these are the physical symptoms by which intense love in the heart sometimes manifests." (Bhakti Rasāmrit Sindhu)

BG 11.15: Arjun said: O Shree Krishna, I witness all the gods and different beings hosted within your cosmic form. I see Brahma seated on the lotus flower (Kamal-Asana); I see Shiva, all the sages, and the divine serpents.

BG 11.16: I see your infinite form in all directions (Disha), with countless arms, stomachs, faces, and eyes. O Lord of the universe, I see your form is the universe itself, I cannot find any beginning, middle, or end in you.

BG 11.17: I see your divine form, bejewelled with a crown, and armed with the club and disc, shining everywhere as the abode of splendour. It is hard to look upon you in the tremendous energy of your effulgence, which is radiating like the sun in all directions.

BG 11.18: I identify you as the supreme immortal Being, the ultimate truth revealed by the scriptures. You are the sustenance of all creation; you are the eternal protector of Sanatan Dharma; and you are the everlasting Supreme Divine Self.

"The goal of all the Vedic mantras is to take us on the path to attain Union with the Divine. He is the primary goal of the study of the Vedas."
(The Kathopanishad 1.2.15)

"The goal of cultivating Vedic knowledge is to attain the Divine. All sacrifices are also meant for pleasing him." (The Śhrīmad Bhāgavatam 1.2.28)

BG 11.19: You are without beginning, middle, or end; your powers are infinite. Your arms are infinite; the sun and the moon are like your eyes, and fire is like your mouth. I see you warming (Tejas) the entire creation by your radiance.

BG 11.20: All the directions as well as space between heaven and earth are all pervaded by you alone. Seeing your astounding and horrifying form, I see the three worlds trembling in fear, O Greatest of all beings.

In this Verse Arjuna is saying, "O Omnipresent Divine, you are all pervading in ten directions, the earth, the sky above, and the space in-between. All living beings are trembling in fear of you."

BG 11.21: All the heavenly gods are taking refuge in your shelter by entering into you. In amazement, some are praising you with folded hands. The great sages and perfected beings are worshiping you with auspicious hymns and generous prayers (Stuti).

BG 11.22: The Rudras, Adityas, Vasus, Sadhyas, Vishvadevas, Ashwini Kumars, Maruts, ancestors, Gandharvas, Yakshas, Asuras, and Siddhas are all witnessing you in wonder.

BG 11.23: O mighty Lord, in adoration of your magnificent form with its many mouths, eyes, arms, thighs, legs, stomachs, and terrifying teeth, all the worlds are terror-stricken, and so am I.

"The Supreme Self (Parmatman) has thousands of heads, thousands of eyes, and thousands of feet. He covers the universe, but is transcendental to it. He resides in all living beings (Jiva), about ten fingers above the navel, in the lotus of the heart." (The Shwetashvatar Upanishad, 3.14)

BG 11.24: O Lord Vishnu, seeing your form touching the sky, effulgent in many colours, with mouths wide open and enormous blazing eyes, my heart is trembling with fear. I have lost all courage and peace of mind.

"Look at the sweetness of the loving interactions between Shree Krishna (Gopal) and his cowherd friends! They play games together, and when Shree Krishna loses the game, he gives a ride to his friends on his back on all fours." (Prem Ras Madirā, Rasiyā Mādhuri, Pada 7)

BG 11.25: Having witnessed your many mouths with your terrible teeth, resembling the violent fire at the time of extinction, I forget where I am and do not know where I go. O Lord of lords, you are the shelter of the universe; please have compassion on me.

BG 11.26-27: I see all the sons of Dhritarashtra, along with their allied kings, including Bheeshma, Dronacharya, Karn, and also the generals from our side, rushing headlong into your fearsome mouths. I also see some with their heads smashed between your terrible teeth.

BG 11.28-29: As many streams of the rivers flowing rapidly into the ocean, so are all these great warriors entering into your blazing mouths. As moths rush with great speed into the fire to perish, so are all these armies entering with great speed into your mouths.

BG 11.30: With your blazing tongues you are licking up the hosts of living beings on all sides and consuming them with your blazing mouths. O Vishnu, you are burning the entire universe with the fierce, all-pervading rays of your effulgence.

BG 11.31: Reveal to me who you are, so ferocious of form. O God of gods, I bow before you; please grant your forgiveness to me. You, who existed before all creation, I wish to know who you are, for I do not comprehend your nature and mechanisms.

BG 11.32: The Supreme Lord said: I am mighty Time and Death (Kala), the source of demolition that comes forth to overpower the worlds. Even without your participation, the warriors grouped in the opposing army shall cease to exist.

BG 11.33: Therefore, ascend and gain honour! Overcome your opponents and enjoy prosperous rulership. These warriors standing in both sides are already eliminated by Me, and you will only be an instrument of my work, O expert archer.

BG 11.34: Dronacharya, Bheeshma, Jayadratha, Karna, and other brave warriors have already been killed by me. So, eliminate them without being concerned. Just fight and you will be victorious over your enemies in battle.

BG 11.35: Sanjay said: Hearing these words of Keshav, Arjun trembled with fright. With palms joined, he bowed before Shree Krishna and spoke in a faltering voice, overwhelmed with fear.

BG 11.36: Arjun said: O Master of the senses (Indiya-Jaya), it is appropriate that the universe rejoices in praising you and is charmed by You. Demons flee fearfully from you in all directions and the souls of perfected saints (Siddhas) bow to you.

BG 11.37: O Greater Self (Maha-Atman), who are even greater than Brahma, the original creator, why should they not bow to you? O limitless One, O Lord of the Devatas, O Refuge of the universe, you are the eternal reality beyond both the manifest and the non-manifest.

"Shree Krishna is the original form of the Supreme Lord. His personality is full of knowledge (Jnana) and Bliss (Ananda). He is the origin of all, but he has no origin. He is the cause of all causes." (Brahma Samhitā 5.1)

BG 11.39: You are Vayu (the lord of wind), Yamraj (the lord of death), Agni (the lord of fire), Varu (the lord of water), and Chandra (the lord moon). You are the creator Brahma, and the great-grandfather of all beings. I offer my salutations unto you a thousand times, again and yet again!

BG 11.40: O Lord of infinite power (Ananta-Virya), my salutations to you from all sides and from deep within! You possess infinite velour and pervade everything, and hence, you are all and everything.

BG 11.41-42: Thinking of you as my friend (Sakha), I arrogantly addressed you as, "O Krishna," "O Yadav," "O my dear friend." I was ignorant of your magnificence, showing negligence and excessive friendliness. And if, zestfully, I treated you with disrespect, while playing, resting, sitting, eating, when alone, or before others—for all that I desire forgiveness.

"I, the Supreme Lord, am in all and everything that exists. There is nothing beyond me and nothing higher than me." (Bhāgavatam 6.4.47)

"The primordial sound 'OM' is a manifestation of the Divine. The Supreme Self is greater than the greatest." (Valmiki Ramayan)
"Divine Self is the Supreme and ultimate Reality that exists." (Manu Smriti 12.122)

BG 11.43: You are the ultimate father (Parma-Pitah) of the entire universe, of all moving and non-moving beings. You are the supreme, worthy of worship and the supreme spiritual master (Adhyatma Guru). When there is no equal to you in all the three worlds, then who can possibly be greater than you, O owner of outstanding power (apratima-prabhava)?

"No-One is equal to Divine, nor is anyone superior to him."
(Shwetashvatar Upanishad 6.8)

BG 11.44: Therefore, O adorable Lord (Priya-Prabhu), bowing sincerely (Pranaam) and prostrating before you, I beg you for your kindness. As a father tolerates his son, a friend forgives his friend, and a lover pardons the beloved, please forgive me for my offences.

BG 11.45: Having seen your divine universal form that I had never witnessed before, I feel great joy. And yet, my mind trembles with fear. Please have compassion on me and again show me your pleasing form, O God of gods (Deva-isha), O abode of the universe (Jagat-Nivasa).

"The divine bliss of God is immensely sweet in all his forms. Yet, there is a progression in it—the bliss of his Dwaraka pastimes is sweet (Madhur), the bliss of his Mathura pastimes is sweeter, and the bliss of his Braj pastimes is the sweetest." (Bhakti Shatak verse 70)

BG 11.46: O thousand-armed one (Sahashra-Baho), though you are the expression of all creation, I wish to see you in your four-armed form (Chatur-Bhuja), carrying the mace and disc, and wearing the crown.

BG 11.47: The Blessed Lord said: Arjun, being pleased (prasanna) with you, by my Yogamaya power, I gave you a vision of my magnificent (Divya-Drashti), unlimited, and primeval cosmic form. No one before you has ever witnessed this.

BG 11.48: Oh best of Kuru warriors, no mortal has ever witnessed what you have. Even the study of Vedas, or the performance of sacrifices, rituals, charity or severe austerities will not bring this experience to mortal beings.

"Without being blessed with the nectar (Amrita) of the grace of the Supreme Lord, nobody can know him." (Yajur Veda)

BG 11.49: Do not be afraid or confused on seeing this horrifying form of mine. Be free from fear (Abhaya) and be with a cheerful heart (Preeta-Manah), witness me once again in my personal form.

BG 11.50: Sanjay said: Having spoken thus, the compassionate son of Vasudev revealed his personal four-armed form again. Then, he further comforted the frightened Arjun by assuming his gentle (two-armed) form (Saumya-Swaroop).

BG 11.51: Arjun said: O Shree Krishna, seeing your gentle human form (two-armed- manusyam rupah), I have regained my composure and my mind is restored to normal.

BG 11.52-53: The Supreme Lord said: This form of mine that you are seeing is exceedingly difficult to witness. Even the heavenly gods are eager to experience IT. Neither by the study of the Vedas, nor by penance, charity, or fire sacrifices, can I be seen as you have seen me.

"The Divine cannot be realised either by spiritual discourses (Satsanga) or through the intellect (Buddhi); nor can he be known by hearing various kinds of teachings." (The Mundakopanishad, 3.2.3)

BG 11.54: O Arjun, by absolute devotion (ananya-Bhakti) alone I can be known just as I am, standing right here for you. Thereby, on receiving my divine vision, O destroyer of enemies, one can attain union with me.

"Devotion alone will unite us with the Divine; devotion alone will help us witness him; devotion alone will help us attain him; Divine is bound by true devotion (Suddha-Bhakti), which is the best of all paths." (Mathar Shruti)

"Uddhav, I reveal myself under the power and love (viriya-prema) of my devotees and I am easily won over by them. But those who do not engage in devotion can never attain me by practicing ashtang yoga, studying Sankhya and other philosophies (Darshanas), performing pious acts (Punya-Karma) and austerities (Tapas), or cultivating renunciation (Sanyasa)." (Bhagavatam 11.14.20)

"I can be only attained through bhakti. Those who engage in my bhakti with faith are very dear to me." (Bhagavatam 11.14.21)

"Without devotion, one can never attain the Divine, no matter how much one endeavours through the practice of ashtang yoga, austerities, knowledge (Jnana), and detachment (Vairajna)." (Ramayan)

BG 11.55: Those who perform all their duties as an instrument of the divine and with divine purpose, who see me as the Supreme Being and behind all the causes and are devoted to me, who are free from attachment (Vairajna), and are free from any form of hatred toward all beings, such devotees certainly attain Me.

"When I walk, I think I am moving around the Lord; when I work, I think I am serving the Lord; and when I sleep, I think I am offering him respect. In this manner, I perform no activity other than that which is offered to him." (Saint and Poet Kabir)

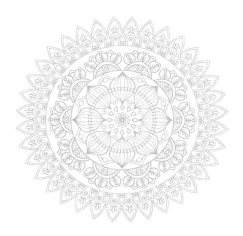

Chapter 12
Yoga of Devotion; Bhakti Yoga

In this chapter Arjuna asks "which one out of the Virata-Bhakti (Saguna Bhakti) or Aksara-bhakti (Nirguna Bhakti) is superior. (B.G. 12.1)

Krishna in the beginning mentions that Saguna-Bhakti is superior as it will lead us to Nirguna-Bhakti. Nriguna Bhakti ultimately leads us to attain union with the Supreme Divine Self. (B.G. 12.2)

Krishna here details various aspects of Bhakti Marga leading the Bhakta to the ultimate of goal of liberation. The Path of Nirguna-Bhakti is also the path of Jnana-Yoga which directly lead us to Supreme Realisation. Further Krishna mentions that one needs to be prepared (Adhikari) to follow the path of Nirguna-Bhakti. (B.G. 12.3 to 5)

First stage of Bhakti is Virata-Upasana or following the Divine in its form with attributes and qualities. Krishna says that such Bhakta will be certainly freed from the Samasara (worldly cycle) by the Lord. (B.G. 12.6 to 8)

Krishna says that, if one even cannot follow the path of virata-bhakti or upasana, he should meditate on any form of the Divine (Istadevata-Upasana) to prepare for nirguna-bhakti.

Krishna further mentions that if the path of meditation is not possible due to the extrovert nature of many, they should perform daily worship (nitya and naimittika) and offerings to the Divine (Iswarap-Arpanam) without the desires of fruits. (B.G. 12.10)

A person full of desires (Vasanas) is driven to perform Karmas born of those desires (Kamya) for the fruits. For those people Krishna says that, "when you receive the fruits of our actions (kamya-karmas), receive them with grace as a divine gift (Prasada) of the Divine. This can be followed with the mantra, "sarva-karma-phalatyagam – all fruits of karmas are blessings of divine." (B.G. 12.11)

These Saguna Upasana Paths also come under Karma Yoga. Karma Yoga prepares one for Saguna Bhakti, which leads one to Nirguna Bhakti and Jnana-Yoga.

Further Krishna details all the characteristics of a Bhakta who has gone through all these steps and attained absolute fulfilment. A Karma Yogi is also a Saguna Bhakta, who sees himself and the Divine as two separate aspects or distinct from himself. This is lower Bhakti, as the Bhakta is not aware of the true nature of the Supreme Lord. This Bhakti is also known as Bheda-Bhakti (devotion of dualistic nature) or Apara-Bhakti (devotion to manifest an aspect of the Divine). Once he pursues the path of Jnana-Yoga and realises the Advaita or Non-Dual, all-pervading nature of the supreme Divine, his bhakti becomes Nirguna-Bhakti (Devotion for formless all-pervading) or Abheda-Bhakti (devotion for non-dual aspect of the Divine) or Para-Bhakti (devotion to the formless unmanifest supreme divine) which the ultimate goal of a Sadhaka. A Nirguna-Bhakta is referred as the Sthita-Prajna (mastered in Equanimity and Self) (B.G. 13.19)

Qualities associated with Para-bhakti	Para-bhakti leads one to be free form:
Maitri - Friendliness	Dvessa - Hatred
Karuna - Compassion	Mamakara -'Mine-ness or I-ness'
Samatvam - Equanimity	Ahankara - Ego
Kshama- Forbearance , forgiveness	Udvega - Anxiety
Santusti - Contentment	Harsha - Excitement
Yata-atmatvam - Self-control	Amarsha - Jealousy
Drdhanishchaya - Firm Self-determination	Bhayam - Fear
Bhakti - Devotion	Apeksa - Dependence and expectation
Bhadrata - Gentleness	Arambha - Selfish action
Suchitvam -Purity	Shoka - Grief
Dakshatvam - Resourcefulness, capabilities	Kanksa - Desire
Udasinatvam - Impartiality	Dvandvas - Pairs of opposites

Krishna concludes this chapter by mentioning that "those who follow these teachings with faith and seek Me as the ultimate goal are very dear to Me (Mama-Priya)."

Yoga of Devotion; Bhakti Yoga

BG 12.1: Arjun asks: Between those who are consistently devoted to Your personal form (Saguna Bhakti) and those who worship the formless Brahman (Nirguna Bhakti), who do You consider to be superior in Yoga?

"The Supreme Self is both with the form (manifest) and formless (unmanifest). Sadhakas of the spiritual path of Bhakti are also of two kinds—devotees of the formless Brahman, and devotees of the Manifest Form of Divine. But the path of worshipping the formless is very difficult."
(Adi Sakarachariya)

BG 12.2: The Divine Lord said: Those who keep their minds focussed on Me and always involve (Nitya-Yukta) in My devotion with steadfast faith, I consider them to be the best of Yogis.

"The knowers of the Truth have stated that there is only one Supreme Divine Self that manifests in three ways in the world—Brahman, Paramatma, and Bhagavan." (The Bhagavatam 1.2.11)

"There is only one Supreme Self. He is contained in everything and everyone." (The Shwetashvatar Upanishad 6.11)

BG 12.3-4: But those who worship the formless aspect (Avyakta, Nirguna) of the Absolute Truth—the eternal, the indefinite, the unmanifest, the all-pervading, the unthinkable, the unchanging, the everlasting, and the immoveable—by restraining their senses (Indriya-Sanniyama) and living in equanimity (Samtva) everywhere, such people, absorbed in the welfare of all living beings, also attain Union with Me.

BG 12.5: For those whose minds are friendly and attracted to the unmanifest (Saguna-Brahma), the path of absolute realisation is not easy to attain. Bhakti of the unmanifest is extremely challenging for manifested beings (Deha-Vadiha – once in the body).

BG 12.6-7: But those who dedicate all their actions (Karma-Bhakti) to Me, observing Me as the Supreme goal, worshiping Me and meditating on Me with wholesome devotion, O Parth, I swiftly lead and liberate them from the ocean of birth and death (Samsara), as their consciousness is united with Me.

BG 12.8: Keep your mind focussed on Me alone and transcend your intellect (Buddhi) to Me. From then, you will always reside in Me, there is no doubt in this.

"Imprisonment in Maya and liberation from it is determined by the mind. If the mind is attached to the worldly objects and desires, one is in bondage; If the mind is detached from the world, one attains liberation." (Bhagavatam 3.25.15)

"Bondage (Bandha) and liberation (Moksha) are decided by the state of the mind." (Panchadashi)

"Our intellect is fastened with wrong knowledge. Though we are eternal souls, we realise ourselves to be the mortal body. Although all the worldly objects are perishable, we believe they will always remain with us, and hence, we actively accumulate them day and night. And though the quest of objects and sensual pleasures only results in misery in the long run, we still chase them in the hope that we will find happiness." (The Bhagavatam 10.40.25)

BG 12.9: Those who are unable to focus their mind steadily on Me, O Arjun, then practice remembering Me with devotion while constantly freeing the mind (Abhyasa-Yogen) from worldly affairs.

BG 12.10: Those who cannot practice remembering Me with devotion, they should try to perform all their Karmas devoted to Me. By performing devotional service to Me, they shall be perfected in preparing for Nirguna Bhakti.

BG 12.11: Those who are even unable to devote their actions to Me, they should try to renounce the fruits of their actions (Niskama-Karma) and remain well established in the Self (Atma).

BG 12.12: Jnana (the cultivation of absolute knowledge) is better than Abhyasa or practice; Meditation (Dhyana) is better than knowledge; Karma-Phala-Tyaga or renouncing the fruits of actions is better than meditation; Renunciation (Sanyasa or Tyaga) instantly follows the Peace (Shanti).

BG 12.13-14: Those devotees are very dear to Me who are free from hatred toward all living beings, who are friendly (Mitra), and compassionate (Karuna). They are free from attachment to possessions and egotism, remain in equanimity (Samatva), in happiness and distress (dvandva), and ever-forgiving (nitya-kshama). They are ever-contented (santosham), steadily united (Satata-Yogi) with Me in devotion, self-controlled (Yata-atma), firm in conviction, and dedicated to Me in mind (Manas) and intellect (Buddhi).

BG 12.15: Those who are not agitating (Udvijate) others and not being agitated by others, who remain equal in pleasure and pain (sukha-dukha), and free from fear and anxiety

(Bhaya-Chinta or Udvega), My such devotees are very dear to Me.

"All the wonderful qualities of the heavenly gods manifest in those who devote themselves to the Supreme Divine Self. But those who do not follow the path of devotion (Bhakti Marga) only keep wandering on the chariot of their mind." (Shreemad Bhagavatam 5.18.12)

BG 12.16: Those who are indifferent to material gain (ana-apeksha), externally and internally pure (Suachi), skilful (Dakshah), who remain calm (Udasina), tranquil (gata-vyatha), and free from selfishness in all accomplishments (Parityagi), such devotees are very dear to Me.

BG 12.17: Those who neither rejoice in mundane pleasures (Raga) nor despair in worldly sorrows (Dwesha), who neither grieve for any loss nor crave for any gain, who renounce both good and evil deeds (shubha-ashubha-parityagi), such persons who practice full devotion are very dear to Me.

BG 12.18-19: Those, who are the same to both friend and enemy (Mitra-Shatru), remain in equanimity in honour and dishonour (Maan-Apamaan), cold and heat (Shita-Ushna), joy and sorrow (Sukha-Dukha), and are free (mukta) from all unfavourable association (Sanga-vivarjita); those who take praise and criticism (stuti-ninda) alike, who are known for silent contemplation (Mauni), content (santushtah) with what comes their way, without attachment to the place of residence, whose intellect is firmly fixed (sthitah) in Me, and who are full of devotion to Me, such persons are very dear to Me.

BG 12.20: Those who honour this nectar of wisdom (jnana-amrita) detailed here, have faith (Sraddha) in Me, and are devoted and absorbed in Me as the Supreme Goal, they are outstandingly dear to Me.

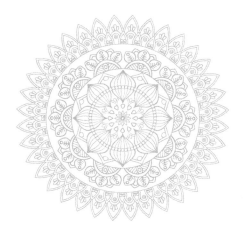

Chapter 13
The Field and Its Knower;
Kshetra Kshetrajna Vibhagha Yoga

Lord Krishna details the nature of Jiva and Karma Yoga in first six chapters, while in the second set of six chapters, He reveals the nature of Ishwara (Supreme Self) and Upasana (Sadhana process to attain union with Supreme Self). These are the steps of sadhana to prepare us for further understanding of Jnana Yoga to recognise the Oneness between the Jiva and Ishwara, which Krishna is revealing the third set of six lessons. In the thirteenth chapter Krishna is introducing six topics:

Kshetram
The entire objective and manifested universe are Kshetram. All that is being experienced by us from the beginningless Prakrati (avyaktam or indescribable) comes under this. It includes mahat (cosmic intellect), ahankara (cosmic ego), the subtle and

gross elements (Pancha-Mahabhutas and their Tanmatras), sense organs of action and perception (Jnanendriyas and Karmendriyas), the mind and its modifications (Manas and Chitta-Vrittis). Krishna also mentions the body as Kshetram, because we generally mistakenly do not see the body as part of the universe.

Kshetrajna

Kshetraja is known to be that conscious principle which illuminates the kshetram. Kshetrajna is none other than the Lord, Ishwara, or Supreme Conscious Self in all that exist. Hence Keshtrajna is the one-all-pervading (sarva-vyapaka) consciousness which is known as Jiva and/or Ishwara.

Jnanam

From the 8th verse to the 12th Krishna discusses some important virtues for preparation of our mind for Atma-Jnana or self-knowledge. These are:- humility, simplicity, non-violence, forbearance, honesty, service to the teacher, purity, steadfastness, self-control, detachment from the objects of senses, free from egoism, total awareness of the suffering in birth and death cycles., dispassion, non-identification with family, house, friends etc., remaining in equanimity in favourable and unfavourable situations, wholesome devotion to the divine, solitude, self-enquiry, and continuously following the path seeking for Self-knowledge.

Jneyam

Krishna further in this chapter reveals the ultimate Truth, which is to be known by great Yogis and Siddhas. It has no beginning and is beyond any end (sat and asat); it is all-pervading and the most subtle, it is impossible for the ignorant (Ajnani) to know and easily known by a wise or realised one (Jnani).

Even though this ultimate truth is Absolute and One, it is the creator, sustainer and destroyer of all. It is the illumination or bliss of consciousness or Chetana which resides in the heart (Hridaya) of each living being. It cannot be known in its purest or subtlest form. It shines or illuminates through the body as Sakshi-Bhava (witnessing awareness) and in the world as Bhava (existence). One needs to realise and experience it as pure Awareness-Existence (Chetana-Deha) by distinguishing it from the body and the world. This sadhana or practice is known as adhyaropa-apavada-prakriya (realising the material existence and the association, and meditating on letting go of attachment to experience - dissociation or detachment). (B.G. 13.13 to 18)

Krishna further mentions that by following this step-by-step process or knowing the gross, subtle and subtlest, will lead the sadhaka ultimately to Him.

Purusha and Prakriti
Krishna mentions that both Purusha and Prakriti neither have any beginning nor have any end. Cosmic Purusha and Prakriti create all and everything. Purusha and Prakriti are opposite in nature. Purusha is conscious, eternal, the ultimate reality and free from change, while Prakriti is inert, changing, and unreal. The body, mind and their activities are fields of the Prakriti while Purusha is merely the witnessing awareness and illuminator of all of those. When the Purusha obtains the body (Kshetra) as the Kshetrajna, it seems to be like a karta (doer), bhokta (consumer) etc. But the Parmatma, the absolute consciousness is ever unaffected, untainted and eternally remains the same. When the Purusha (Kshetrajna) identifies with the body and its gunas, then, all the limitations (ajnana, asmita, avidya, etc) and the consequent sufferings arise. One

who has this discriminative knowledge (Viveka-Jnana) and awareness of Purusha and Prakriti attains immortality. (B.G. 13. 20 to 24)

In this chapter Krishna further sums up the teachings and reveals the practice (Sadhanam) and the fruits of sadhana (phalam). The wiseman (Jnani) is the one who remains established in the Ultimate Self (Parmatma), which is the same in all and everywhere. The Atman is free from all the Karmas (actions) and remains unaffected by their cause and reactions or fruits like the Akasha or space (Akasha) or the light (Jyoti). The Atman or Self is the illuminator of all and everything as well as the foundation of the whole universe. The ultimate truth is, "there is nothing other than the Atman that exists in Reality." One who has realised this knowledge and remains well established in this Cosmic Awareness becomes Brahma Itself (Ahama-Brahmasmi) and attains the ultimate goal of liberation (Kaivalya). (B.G. 13. 25 to 35)

To attain this knowledge, one needs to purify the mind through Karma Yoga, gain knowledge through self-enquiry (Samkhya-Yoga) and ultimately unite the mind and awareness in the Supreme Self through meditation (Dhyana Yoga).

The Field and Its Knower; Kshetra Kshetrajna Vibhagha Yoga

BG 13.1: Arjun spoke, "O Keshav, I seek to know about the prakriti and the purusha, and what are the kshetra and kshetrajja? I also wish to know what is True Knowledge, and what is the goal of this knowledge?

Prakriti – the manifest or material nature
Purusha – the Jiva or Living Being, Consciousness
Kshetram – the field of activities like body
Kshetrajna – knower or the awareness of the fields of activities
Jnanam – Knowledge
Iccha – Wish, desire

BG 13.2: Shree Bhagavan said: O Arjun, this body (sharira) is known as kshetra (the field of activities), and the one who knows (awareness) the body is known as kshetrajja (the awareness of the field) by the sages who recognise the truth about these two.

BG 13.3: O offspring of Bharat, I am also the knower of all the individual fields of activity. The knowing of the body as the field of activities, and the soul (Jiva or Atma) and Divine (Iswara or Parmatman) as the knowers of the field, this 'I' is known to be the True Knowledge.

Here in a simple way, "Knowing of the self, the Supreme Divine, the body, and the distinction amongst these, is true knowledge."

BG 13.4: Listen, I will reveal to you about that field and its nature as well. I will also reveal how change takes place within this field, from what it was created, who the knower of the field of activities is, and what his powers are.

BG 13.5: Great Rishis have sung the truth about the field and the knower of the field in manifold ways. It has been mentioned in various hymns of Vedas, and especially revealed in the Brahma Sūtra, with comprehensive logic and conclusive evidence.

According to the Vedas, "truth is one, but the wise speak it in many ways, ekam-sat-vipra-bahuda-vandanti."

BG 13.6: The Kshetra or body is constituted of the five major elements (pancha-maha-bhutas), the ego (ahamkara), the intellect (Buddhi), the unmanifest primordial matter (apara-prakriti or avyaktam), the eleven senses (pancha-jnenendiryas, pancha-karmendriyas and manas), and the five objects of the senses (tanmatras).

BG 13.7: Desire (Iccha) and aversion (dwesha), pleasure (sukha) and pain (dukha), the body (sharira), awareness (chetana), and the will (dhriti)—of all these are comprised the field (Kshetra) and its modifications.

According to Vedic teachings the body is the instrument or vehicle of the soul and the body undergoes six transformations until death:
- **asti** (coming into existence in the womb)
- **jayate** (birth)
- **vardhate** (growth)
- **viparinamate** (reproduction)
- **apakshiyate** (withering with age)
- **vinashyati** (death).

BG 13.8-12: These five verses describe the virtues, habits, behaviours, and attitudes that purify one's heart, mind and life and illuminate it with the light of knowledge (jnana-jyoti).

These virtues are:

- ❏ **Amanitvam** - humility
- ❏ **Adambhitvam** - freedom from hypocrisy
- ❏ **Ahimsa** - Non-violence
- ❏ **Kshantih** - forgiveness
- ❏ **Aarjavam** - simplicity
- ❏ **Achariya Upasanam** - service of the Guru
- ❏ **Shaucham** - purity or cleanliness of the body and mind
- ❏ **Sthairyam** - steadfastness or stability
- ❏ **Indriya-Astheshu-Atma-vinigraha** - self-control or discipline towards objects of sense
- ❏ Vairagyam - detachment or dissociation
- ❏ **Anahankarah** - absence of egoism
- ❏ **Jnana-Janma-Mrityu-Jara-Vyadhi-Dukha-dosha** - Knowing of birth, death, old age, disease, suffering, and faults
- ❏ **Anudarshanam-Asaktih** - awareness of non-dependence
- ❏ **Anabhishvangah** - absence of attachment or cravings towards children (putra), dara (spouse), home (griha) etc.
- ❏ **Nitya-sama-chttatvam** - continual equanimity of mind in the desirable (ishta) and undersirable (anishta) situations
- ❏ **Upapattishu mayi-ananya-yogen** - desire and effort to attain absolute union in Divine
- ❏ **Bhakti** - devotion
- ❏ **Avyabhicharini-Vivikta** - continual solitary

- **Aratih-jana-sansadi** - aversion from the mundane society
- **Adhyatma-jnana-nityama** - continually seeking for true spiritual knowledge
- **Tattva-Jnana-Darshnam** - effort to attain knowledge of absolute truth.

Krishna says that what is contrary to these virtues is known to be Ajnana or ignorance.

jaba main thā taba hari nathīn, ab hari hai, main nāhīn
prem galī ati sankarī, yā men dwe na samāhīn   (Saint Kabir)

"When 'I' existed, the Divine was not there; now the Divine exists but 'I' do not. The path of divine love is very narrow; it cannot accommodate both 'I' and God."

BG 13.13: Now, I will reveal to you what is really there to be known, and by knowing which, one attains immortality (amritvam). It is the beginningless (Anadi) Brahman, which exists beyond all that exist (sat) and that which does not exist (asat).

BG 13.14: The hands and feet, eyes, heads, and faces of the Divine are all and everywhere. His ears too are in all places, as He is all-pervading in the universe.

BG 13.15: Though He identifies all sense-objects, yet He is free of the senses and their objects. He is not attached to anything, and yet He is the sustainer of all. Though He is free from attributes, yet He is the witness of the three modes (tri-gunas) of material nature.

BG 13.16: He exists within (antar) and beyond (bahir) all living beings (jiva), the moving (chala) and not moving (achala) beings. He is subtle (sukshma), and He is incomprehensible. He seems to be beyond the reach, but He is also very near within all.

"The Supreme Brahman does not walk, and yet He walks; He is far, but He is also near. He exists inside everything, but He is also outside everything." (Ishopanishad)

BG 13.17: He is indivisible, yet He seems to be differed amongst living beings (Jivatma). Know the Supreme Being (Parmatman) to be the Creator, Sustainer, and Annihilator of all beings.

"The various aspects of creation—time, karma, the natures of individual living beings, and the material elements of creation—all these are the Supreme Lord Shree Krishna Himself. There is nothing in existence other than Him." (Shrimad Bhagavad 2.5.14)

BG 13.18: He is the source of light (jyoti) in all that shines or stars and is exclusively beyond the darkness (tamas) of ignorance (avidya). He is the knowledge, the object of knowledge, and the goal of knowledge. He dwells within the hearts of all living beings.
"The Divine makes all things luminous. It is by His luminosity that all luminous objects spring light." (Kathopanishad 2.2.15)

"By His radiance, the sun and moon become luminous." (Vedas)

BG 13.19: I have revealed to you the nature of the field, the significance of knowledge, and the object of knowledge. Only My devotees can realise this in authenticity, and by doing so, they attain My divine nature.

"Those who practice bhakti toward the Supreme Divine Being, giving up all material desires, are freed from the cycle of life and death." (Mundakopanishad 3.2.1)

"Those who have steady bhakti toward God and identical bhakti toward the Guru, in the hearts of such saintly persons, by the grace of God the meanings of the Vedic scriptures are automatically revealed." (Shwetashvar Upanishad 6.23)

BG 13.20: The Prakriti (material nature) and Purusha (the individual soul) are both ever-existing (Anadi). Also all transformations of the body and the three modes of nature (tri-gunas) are created by material energy.

According to Paramatma Sandarbh, "The soul is a fragment of the jiva shakti (life force) of the Divine."

BG 13.21: In the process of creation, the material energy is responsible for cause and effect (Karya-Karan) while in the subject of experiencing pleasure and pain (sukha-dukha), the individual soul is known to be responsible.

"The world is pervaded by the Divine. It creates an illusion (Maya), which is unreal, but brings misery to the living being. This is just like if someone's head is being cut in the dream, the suffering will continue until the person wakes up and stops dreaming." (Ramayana)

BG 13.22: When the purusha (individual soul) contained in Prakriti (the material energy) desires to enjoy the outcomes the three gunas, attachment to them becomes the cause of its birth in superior and inferior wombs (sat-asat-yoni).

BG 13.23: Iswara or the Supreme Self also resides in the body. He is known to be the Witnessing Awareness (Sakshi), the All-pervading, the Supporter, Transcendental Enjoyer, the ultimate Regulator, and the Paramatma (Supreme Soul).

Manduka Upanishad States, "Two birds are seated in the nest (heart) of the tree (the body) of the living form. They are the jivatma (individual self) and Paramatma (Supreme Self). The jivatma has its back toward the Paramatma, and is busy enjoying the fruits of the tree (the results of the karmas it receives while residing in the body). When a sweet fruit comes, it feels happy; when a bitter fruit comes, it feels sad. The Paramatma is a friend of the jivatma, but He does not interfere; He simply sits and witnesses. If the jivatma can only turn around to the Paramatma, all its miseries will come to an end."

BG 13.24: Those who know the truth about Parmatman, the individual soul or Jiva, Prakriti, and the interaction of the tri-gunas will become free from birth. They will be liberated regardless of their present circumstance.

Swetashwar Upanishad states that "There are three aspects in creation—the ever-changing material nature (Prakriti), the unchangeable souls (Atman), and the Supreme Self (Iswara). Ignorance (Vidya) or not knowing of this is the cause of bondage of the soul, while knowledge of this helps in becoming free from Maya."

BG 13.25: Some try to identify the Supreme Self within their hearts through meditation (Dhyana Yoga Marga), and others try to do so through the cultivation of knowledge (Jnana Yoga

Marga), while others strive to attain that realisation by the path of action (Karma Yoga Marga).

BG 13.26: There are also others who are ignorant of these spiritual paths (Adhyatma Marga), but they hear of this knowledge from others and begin worshipping the Divine. By such devotion to hearing from saints, they too can gradually cross over the ocean of birth and death (Samsara-Mukti). (Satsanga Marga)

King Parikshit asked Shukadev, "How can we purify the undesirable thoughts, feelings and emotions from our hearts, such as lust, anger, greed, envy, hatred, etc.?"

Shukadev replied: "Parikshit! Simply hear the descriptions of the divine Names, Forms, Activities or Divine Stories, Virtues, Abodes, and about Divine Maharishis from a Rishi or saint. This will naturally cleanse the heart of the unwanted impurities of endless lifetimes."
(Bhagavatam 1.2.17)

BG 13.27: O best of the Bharatas, whatever moving or unmoving being (sthavara-jangaman) you witness, realise it to be a combination of the field of activities and the knower of the field (kshetra-kshetrajna samyoga).
BG 13.28: They alone truly realise, who perceive the Paramatma (Supreme Self) accompanying the soul in all beings, and who know both to be eternal in this perishable body.

"Supreme Divine is One. He dwells in the hearts of all living beings. He is omnipresent. He is the Supreme Soul of all souls." (Shwetashvatar Upanishad 6.11)

"Supreme Self is contained inside all living beings as the Witness and the Master." (Bhagavatam 10.86.31)

"The Supreme Lord Ram is eternal and beyond everything. He resides in the hearts of all living beings." (Ramayan)

BG 13.29: Those, who see the Divine as the Supreme Self equally present everywhere and in all living beings, are free from the lower fields of their mind. By this, they attain the supreme goal.

BG 13.30: They alone know the truth, who know that all actions (of the body) are performed by material nature, while the conscious soul actually is not doing anything.

The Tantra Bhagavat mentions: "The knowing of the body as Atman or being and the ego of being the doer (karta-ahamkara) trap the soul in the samsara of life and death."

Maharishi Vasishth initiated Ram: "Ram, while performing actions, externally employ Yourself as if the fruits of actions depend upon You; but internally, know Yourself to be the non-doer."

BG 13.31: When they see the different variety of living beings located in the same material nature, and know all of them to be born from it, they attain the supreme realisation.

All living being are rooted in the same Reality—the soul, which is a part of the Divine, seated in a body, which is made from the same material energy.

BG 13.32: The Supreme Self is immortal, without beginning, and free from any material qualities (nirgunatvat), O son of

Kunti. Even though seated within the body (sharira sthita), It neither acts (akarta), nor is It tainted by material energy.

BG 13.33: Voidness (Akasha) holds everything within it, but being subtle, does not get adulterated by what it holds. Similarly, though the consciousness pervades the body, still the soul is not affected by the attributes of the body.

BG 13.34: Just as one sun illumines the entire solar system, so does the individual soul illumine the entire body.

"If we divide the tip of a hair into a hundred parts, and then divide each part into a further hundred parts, we will get the size of the soul. These souls are innumerable in number." (Shwetashvatar Upanishad 5.9)

"The soul seated in the heart spreads its consciousness throughout the field of the body." (Vedanta Darshan 2.3.25)

BG 13.35: Those who perceive the difference between the body and the knower of the body, and the process of liberation from material nature through the eyes of knowledge, attain the ultimate goal.

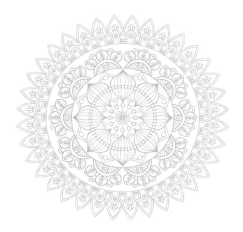

Chapter 14
The Yoga of Gunas;
Gunatraya Vibhaga Yoga

In the previous chapter Krishna mentioned that the association of the Gunas of the Prakriti are responsible for rebirth and the cycle of Samsara. In this chapter Krishna details the concept of the Gunas and how to transcend in order to free ourselves from this association with the Gunas.

Krishna begins this chapter by praising the Atma-Jnana for Arjuna's attention. The supreme knowledge of Reality or the Divine leads one to the ultimate goal of liberation. By realising this wisdom, one attains the nature and qualities of the Divine Itself and becomes free from birth cycles or Samasara.

Krishna reveals that with the blessings of the Supreme Consciousness (Parmatman), the Prakriti gives birth to this universe. Thus Prakriti and Parmatman are the universal parents of all living and non-living beings of originate.

The three Gunas are Sattva, Rajas, and Tamas. These gunas are born of the Prakriti and are responsible for the human bondage and cycle of birth and death.

Guna	Sattva	Rajas	Tamas
Lakshanam	Prakastmakam	Ragamatmakam	Mohanatamakam
Qualities	Illumination, light	Delusion	Attachment
Bandhanaprakara	Jnanasanga	Karmasanga	Pramadsanga
Mode of association	Knowledge	Action or activity	Inertia or inaction
Lingam	Jnanavriddhi	Karmavriddhi	Pramavriddhi
Sign of Predominance	Increase in Knowledge	Increase in activity	Increase in Inertia or Inaction
Gati	Urdhvagati	Madhyagati	Adhogati
Move towards	Towards higher lokas	To middle lokas	To lower lokas
Phalam	Punya and Jnana	Dukham and Lobha	Ajnana and Moha
Fruits	Bliss and Wisdom	Suffering and greed	Ignorance and delusion

All beings have these three gunas, but they differ from each other because of the predominance and combination of the gunas over one and another. It is possible to change the proportions and predominance of the gunas through sadhana.

Transcending the Gunas is a Sadhana and/or Vidya all of its own. The Purusha or soul by its eternal and absolute nature is known to be already beyond the gunas (gunatita). The body or kshetra is subject to the gunas and their transformations. Because of avidya or ignorance, we identify ourselves with the body, which is why the Self or Purusha seems to have the gunas in appearance. By means of Atma-Jnana, Sadhana will develop the discrimination to realise the gunatita pusursha as Reality of the Self. By means of this realisation and wisdom, one attains liberation from cycle of birth and death of Samsara. This is the ultimate liberation of Kaivalya.

In verse 21 Arjuna asks Krishna to reveal the characteristics of Gunatita and the Sadhana process to achieve this.

According to Krishna, Gunatita is one who is free from the Prakriti and its modifications by means of Tri-Gunas. He is free from I-ness (Asmita) and My-ness (Ahamkara) in the manifest world. He sees the modifications of gunas objectively as the witness without reacting to them or without being influenced by them. He remains in equanimity and unaffected in the opposite experiences (dvandva) of pain-pleasure, praise-criticism, honour-dishonour etc. These opposites are outcomes of the Prakriti and gunas. Being Wholesome or One, the Self does not seek for anything and remains free from all forms of selfish activities and desires. These qualities are equal with the Jnani, Yogi, Sthita-Prajna and Para-bhakta.

Krishna concludes this chapter by reminding us of Bhakti as the Sadhana Path to achieve this ultimate goal. It is mentioned that by grace of the Divine, one meets a Guru. By blessings of a Guru one attains knowledge which leads the sadhaka to the state of Gunatita. By means of Bhakti one becomes Adhikari (eligible and suitable) to attain oneness with qualities of Brahman (Gunati-tatvam) which is immortal, eternal and absolute bliss (sat-chit-ananda).

The Yoga of Gunas;
Gunatraya Vibhaga Yoga

BG 14.1: Shree Bhagavan said: Once again I shall explain to you the supreme wisdom (Param-Jnana), the best of all knowledge (Jnanam); by knowing which, all the Munis or great saints attained the Siddhis or ultimate perfection.

BG 14.2: Those who take shelter (sharanagati or upashritya) in this wisdom will be united with Me. They will be free from birth at the time of creation and will not be destroyed at the time of dissolution (Maha-pralaya).

BG 14.3-4: Prakriti is the womb (Yoni) of all the material existence. I impregnate it with the Jiva or Atman (individual souls), and in this way all living beings (sarve-jiva) are born. O son of Kunti, for all species of life that are created, the Prakriti is the womb (Garbha), and I am the seed-giving Father (Bija-Pradah-Pita).

"In the womb of the material energy (Prakriti-Garbha) the Supreme Divine impregnates the souls. Then, stimulated by the karmas of the individual souls, the material nature creates suitable life forms for them."
(Shrimad Bhagavatam 3.26.19)

BG 14.5: O mighty-armed Arjun, the material energy consists of three gunas (primordial qualities)—sattva (goodness), rajas (passion), and tamas (inertia). These qualities bind the eternal soul to the perishable body.

BG 14.6: Amongst these, sattva guna, the quality of goodness, being purest (nirmal) of the three, is illuminating (prakasha) and full of well-being or peacefulness (anamayam). O sinless one, it binds (bandha) the soul by desires for happiness (sukha) and knowledge (jnana).

BG 14.7: O Arjuna, rajo guna has the nature of passion. It ascends from worldly desires (trishna), affection and associations (sanga), and binds the soul through desires for the fruits of actions (karma-phala).

BG 14.8: O Arjuna, tamo guna, which is born of ignorance (Ajnana), is the cause of illusion (moha) as the recognition of the body as the Self or Atma. It deludes all living beings through negligence (Pramada), laziness (Alasya), and sleep (Nidra).

BG 14.9: Sattva binds one towards happiness (Sukha); rajas binds the soul toward actions (Karma); and tamas clouds wisdom and binds one to delusion and lack of drive towards actions.

BG 14.10: The Sattva or goodness predominates over rajas or passion (rajas) and tamas or ignorance sometimes, O offspring of Bharat. While rajas dominates sattva and tamas sometimes. Other times tamas dominates sattva and rajas.

In this Krishna is revealing that one of the three Gunas is dominating the other two, depending on the state of body, mind, thoughts, samaskaras, karmas, desires etc. The Sattva guna seeks for peace, contentment, generosity, calmness, care, helpfulness and serenity. The Rajo guna drives one towards passion, action, ambition, agitation, and sense of pleasures and material fulfilment. The Tamo guna is characterised by sleep, laziness, hatred, selfishness, anger, resentment, violence, doubt, illusion, and lack of motivation.

BG 14.11: In the Sattva Guna manifestation of all the gates of the body (deha-dwara) are illumined by knowledge (jnana-prakasha).

BG 14.12: In the predominance of the Rajas Guna the mode of passion, O Arjun, the symptoms of greed, exertion for worldly gain, restlessness, and craving develop.

BG 14.13: O Arjun, ignorance, inertia, negligence, and delusion are the dominant signs of the Tamo Guna.

These gunas even influence our spiritual journey. When sattva is active, we find so much love and gratitude for all that we are receiving from nature, the divine, guru and friends and family and are naturally driven to believe in the divine. Rajo Guna is driven by passion and fruits of actions, which also develops some divine intentions and gratitude, but due to material desires and priorities, we struggle to find actual time and energy to follow the path of divinity. While the Tamo Guna is active, we are deep down in ignorance, selfish desires, and lack the drive to do anything. Here we totally lose faith in the divine or any form of goodness in life and even wonder why we should waste time in Sadhana.

BG 14.14-15: One who leaves the body with predominance of sattva will reach the pure abodes of the learned or wise (uttam-vidyabham). Those who die with dominance of the Rajas are born among people driven by actions (karma), while those dying while Tamas is active take birth in the lower nature beings (mudha-yoni).

BG 14.16: The fruit of actions performed in the Sattva guna bring pure or soothing results (Nirmala phala). Actions done in the Rajas Guna or under the quality of passion result in pain (dukham), while actions performed in the tamas guna or quality of ignorance result in darkness.

BG 14.17: From the Sattva arises knowledge, from the Rajas arises greed, and from the tamas arise negligence and delusion.

BG 14.18: Those situated in the Sattva Vritti (pure thoughts) rise upward; those in the Rajas Vritti stay in the middle; and those in the Tamas Vritti go downward.

"Those who are in Sattva guna *reach the higher heavenly abodes; those who are in* Rajo guna *return to the earth planet; and those who remain in* Tamo guna *go to the lower planes of existence; while those who are transcendental to the Gunas (Gunatitah) attain Me." (Bhagavatam 11.25.22)*

BG 14.19: A wise person realises that all actions are performed only under the modes of three gunas. There are no any other means of action. Those wise souls know the divine as gunatitah (transcendental to the modes of gunas) and surely attain the absolute divine nature or quality.

BG 14.20: By transcending the Gunas of Prakriti or material nature associated with the body, one becomes free from birth, death, old age, and misery, and attains immortality (Amritvam).

BG 14.21: Arjuna asked: What are the characteristics of those who have transcended the three gunas, O Lord? How do they act? How do they transcend the Gunas and liberate from the operations of the gunas?

BG 14.22-23: Shri Bhagavan replied: O Arjuna, The persons who have transcended the three gunas neither dislike illumination (fruit of sattva), nor activity (arise out of rajas), nor even delusion (as a result of tamas), when these are abundantly present. Nor do they desire for them when they are absent. They remain neutral to the Gunas and are not disturbed by them and their manifestations. Know that it is only the gunas that act, they stay established in the self, and remain free from disturbances.

BG 14.24-25: Those who remain balanced (sama-bhava) in happiness and distress (sukha-dukha); who are established in the self (atma-nistha); who see a clod, a stone, and a piece of gold as of equal value in existence; who remain in equanimity (sama-tulya) amidst pleasant (priya) and unpleasant (apriya) events; who are wise and see both criticism (ninda) and praise (sanstusti) with equanimity; who remain centred in balance (sama-bhava) in honour and dishonour (mana-apamana); who treat both friend and enemy alike; and who have renounced (parityagah) all establishments (sarva-arambha)– they are known to have risen above the three gunas (gunatitah).

BG 14.26: Those who serve me with absolute or pure devotion (bhakti-yoga) rise above the three gunas or Prakriti and rise to the level of Brahman (Brahma-Bhuyaya).

Sage Ved Vyasa mentions in the Padma Purana that "the scriptures refer to the Divine or Ishwara as nirguna (free from qualities of gunas). This means that the Divine is free from material attributes or manifest nature. But the divine Self (Parmatman) is not devoid of qualities—he possesses infinite divine attributes (Divya-Guna)."

BG 14.27: I am the source of the formless Brahman, the immortal (amritam) and imperishable (avyayasya), of eternal dharma (Shasavat Dharma), and of never-ending divine bliss (sukha-aikantikasya).

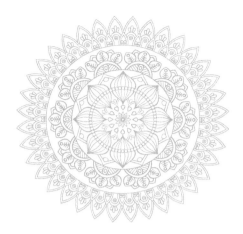

Chapter 15
Yoga of the Supreme Spirit;
Purushottama Yoga

In chapter 13 and 14 Lord Krishna has revealed the non-dualistic (Advaita) of Jiva and Ishwara.

Krishna begins this chapter by comparing the vastness and endless nature of Samsara with the mighty ashvattha tree. Like this tree, the samsara is vast, multi-branched, well-rooted and not easily destructible. It is also mysterious in nature. Jiva is caught in the illusion of samsara and seems like helplessly struggling to free itself.

Further Krishna teaches us following techniques to liberate ourselves from miseries of samsara by the following means:

1. **Vairajna** – developing detachment from samsara by knowing its binding and changing nature or illusion and freeing the mind from worldly desires.

2. **Know Brahma** or the supreme Self as the ultimate cause of everything.

Following these two practices, Krishna points out the qualifications (adhikara-guna), which are:

❏   Sakshi and Samabhava – Awareness and equanimity in the pairs of opposites (sukha-dukha – pleasant-painful, maan-apmaan – honour-dishonour, Priya-apriya – favourable-unfavourable).

❏   Veda-Jnana-Shraddha – faith in Vedic teachings and commitment in Jnana-Chintan or Enquiry for True Knowledge.

Krishna mentions that the Brahma or Supreme Self is Supreme and the Source of all that is manifest, and unmanifest. The Supreme Self is not illuminated by anything as it is the self-effulgent consciousness which illuminates everything else. One who attains this knowledge and realisation does not return to samsara again.

Here Krishna reveals that Brahma or the Supreme Self alone manifests in the form of Jiva (Individual self) and Jagat (manifest world). This clearly means that the Supreme Self is within us all and everything and there is no need to go anywhere else to search for That.

The Jiva, the consciousness in every living being, is the expression of the Supreme Self, Brahma only. At the time of death (mrityu-kala), the Jiva alone takes the mind and sense organs from one body to another body. Jiva only experiences everything by means of the sense organs. The Supreme Self alone is expressing in the form of every life and their functions. Ajnanis because of the delusion of 'I-ness or I Do' see body, mind and sensory objects as ultimate reality. The Realised Ones (Jnanis) with pure mind (Nirmala manas) know this Supreme nature of all-pervading Parmatman.

Further Krishna details the ultimate truth and qualities of the Parmatman or Supreme Consciousness. The light of the sun and the moon, as well as the heat is mere expression of Parmatman. The Supreme Self sustains life in the form of the sunlight (roshani) and moonlight (chandani). Parmatman digests food in the form of digestive fire (jatharagni). Consciouness alone is behind the fields of wisdom, memory, thinking and realisations etc. He is the creator, author (Rachiyata) and the teachings (Siksha) of the Vedas as well as the Knower of the Vedas.

Shri Bhagawan further reveals the true nature of Brahman. Parmatman, in the manifest form (manifest universe) is known as the Kshara-purusha. As the unmanifest universe (apara-maya) the same Parmatman is known as akshara-purusha. Both aspects of the purusha are relative. There is also the absolute consciousness superior beyond the above two purushas known as uttama-purusha. Because of its superiority it is also known as Paramatma or Purushottama. This Brahma is the eternal, free from attributes and everything exists only because of It.

Krishna concludes that this Knowledge or Vidya is the means of the absolute fulfilment (atma-santusthi). One who knows the ultimate reality of the Purushottama becomes all-knowing and absolutely fulfilled or content.

Yoga of the Supreme Spirit; Purushottama Yoga

BG 15.1: Shri Bhagavan said: The wise refer an eternal ashvatth (Peepal or sacred fig) tree with its roots growing upward (udharva-moola) and branches downward (adhah-sakham). Each of the tree's leaves is like a Vedic hymn, and one who knows the secret of this tree is the knower of the Vedas.

"The ashvatth tree, with its roots upward and branches downward is eternal." (Kathopanishad 2.3.1)
"Those who know this tree with its roots upward and branches downward know that death cannot finish them." (Taittiriya Aranyak 1.11.5)

BG 15.2: The branches of the tree extend upward and downward, nourished by the three Gunas, with the objects of the senses (indriya-visaya) as tender buds. The roots of the tree hang downward, initiating the flow of karma in the human form. Beneath, the roots are causing Karmas in the human world.

BG 15.3-4: The true form of this tree cannot be perceived in this world, neither its beginning nor end, nor its continued existence. But this deep-rooted ashvatth tree of samsara must be cut down with a strong axe of detachment (Vairajna). Then one must look for the base of the tree, which is the Supreme

Self, from whom sprung out the activity of the universe a long time ago. One will not return to this worldly field after taking refuge in the Supreme Self.

Upasana – Asanga follows Sanga:- dissociation or detachment from the worldly objects and negative association should be followed by association or connection (sanga, satsanga) with the Higher Self. This verse advises us to use the Vairajna and Asanga as the tool to disconnect or dissociate from negative karma, samaskaras and worldly objects of suffering. Then seek for the central root, which is the Supreme Self in the case of living beings, and connect with That to attain liberation.

BG 15.5: Those who are free from egotism and delusion (maan-moha), who have overcome the evil of attachment (sanga-dosha), who dwell continually in the Self and Divine, who are free from the desires of sensory pleasure, and are beyond the dualities (dvandva-vimukti) of pleasure and pain (sukha-dukha), such liberated beings (mukta-jiva) attain My Eternal Abode.

"This impermanent world created from the material energy is only one part of creation. The other three parts are the eternal Abode of the Divine that is beyond the phenomenon of life and death." (Purush Suktam Mantra 3)

BG 15.6: The Supreme Abode of the Field of Consciousness does not need to be illuminated by the sun or the moon or the fire. The Consciousness or Parmatman is self-illuminating and the source of all and everything. One who will reach this abode, will not return to the material world again.

BG 15.7: The living beings (jiva-bhuta) in this material world (jiva-loka) are My eternal fragmental parts (anshah). They are bound by material nature (prakriti-gunah), they are deluded or caught with the six senses (shata-indriyas) including the mind.

Swansh: All that exists is a fraction of the Supreme Self.
Vibhinnansh: All the living beings or souls separated from the Supreme Self by the field of Gunas, Karma, Samaskara etc. These manifest from the Jiva-Shakti. These are divided in three categories:

Nitya Siddha: The Self-realised souls residing in Divine Consciousness.
Sadhan Siddha: Attaining the Divine Nature or Realisation through Sadhana.
Nitya Baddha: Bhuta-Jiva or living beings bounded in material realm or Samsara.

BG 15.8: As the wind (Vayu) carries fragrance (sugandha) from place to place, so does the living being carry the mind and senses with it, when it moves from an old body to a new one.

BG 15.9: Using the sensory cognition of the ears (shrotra), eyes (Chakshu), skin (sparsha), tongue (rasa), and nose (ghrana), which are connected around the mind (manas), the living being consumes the sensory objects.

BG 15.10: The ignorant (Vimudha) cannot see the eternal soul as it resides in the body, and enjoys sensory objects; nor do they perceive it when it departs the body. But those with the eyes of wisdom (jnana-chakshu) know the Truth of Atma-Nityam (eternity of soul).

BG 15.11: Endeavouring yogis (Yatnah-Yogi) are also able to realise the soul treasured in the body. However, those with impure minds (akrita-atmanah) cannot perceive this reality, even if they attempt to do so.

Alexis Carrel, in his book, Man the Unknown, states: "Our mind has a natural tendency to reject the things that do not fit into the frame of scientific or philosophical beliefs of our time. After all, scientists are only human. They are saturated with the prejudices of their environment and epoch. They willingly believe that facts which cannot be explained by current theories do not exist. At present times, scientists still look upon telepathy and other metaphysical phenomena as illusions. Evident facts having an unorthodox appearance are suppressed."

BG 15.12: Know that I am like the illumination (teja) of the sun that brightens (prakashah) the entire solar system. The radiance of the moon and the brightness of the fire also come from Me.

BG 15.13: Pervading the earth, I nourish all living beings (bhuta-jiva) with My energy (ojas). Becoming the moonlight (somah), I nourish all plants (oshadhyah) with the juice of life (rasa-atmaka).

BG 15.14: It is I who take the form of the fire of digestion (jatharagni) in the stomach of all living beings, and association with the inhalation and exhalation of vital energies (prana-apana), to digest and assimilate the four kinds of foods.

The four types of food:

1. Bhojya - Foods that are chewed, like bread, fruits, vegetables etc.
2. Peya - Foods which we swallow or drink like water, juice, milk etc.
3. Koshya - Foods that are sucked, like sugarcane.
4. Lehya - This includes foods that are licked, such as honey etc.

BG 15.15: I am seated in the hearts of all living beings, and I am the memory (smriti), knowledge (Jnana), as well as forgetfulness (apohanam). I alone am the ultimate aim to be known by all the Vedas, I am the author of the Vedanta, and I am the knower of the essence and meaning of the Vedas.

"From the Divine alone, the knowledge of the living being arises, and by the Divine Maya that knowledge is stolen away." (Bhagavatam 11.22.28)

BG 15.16: There are two kinds of beings (dvi-purusha) in creation (loka), the kshar (mortal) and the akshar (immortal). The mortals are all beings in the material world (bhuta-jagat). The immortals are the liberated beings.

BG 15.17: The Supreme Divine Self (Uttama-Purusha) is in the foundation and beyond all that, He is the everlasting Supreme Soul. He pervades the three worlds (loka-tryam) as the invariable regulator and supports all living beings.

BG 15.18: I am transcendental to the mortal world of matter, and the eternal soul; hence I am admired in the Vedas and the Smritis, as the Supreme Divine Self.

BG 15.19: Those who know Me without any doubt as the Supreme Conscious Self truly have wholesome knowledge. O Arjuna, those who know this worship Me with their whole being.

"The knowers of the Truth have affirmed that there is only one Supreme Self that manifests in three aspects in the world—Brahman, Paramatma, and Bhagavan." (Shrimada Bhagavad 1.2.11)

"As Brahman, the infinite energies of the Divine are all latent. He purely displays eternal knowledge and bliss." (Bhakti Shatak verse 22)

"As Paramatma, the Supreme Divine manifests His Form, Name, and Virtues. But He does not engage in Leelas, nor does He have association with any." (Bhakti Shatak verse 23)

BG 15.20: I have revealed this most secret knowledge of the Vedic scriptures to you, O sinless Arjuna. By understanding this, a person attains enlightenment, and fulfils all that is to be accomplished.

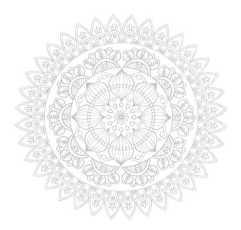

Chapter 16
The Field and Its Knower;
Kshetra Kshetrajna Vibhagha Yoga

In the previous few chapters Lord Krishna has revealed the Jnana-Yoga as the important path and means to liberation. In chapter 16 and 17 He reveals the values or virtues to be followed by the seekers of liberation. These virtues are to prepare a sadhaka to attain and experience the absolute truth or reality. They prepare the mind to be ready and eligible (adhikari) to receive the Absolute Wisdom known as Atma-Jnana. It is said that Vedic wisdom is a Pramana (source of direct knowledge) for the mind that is ready to receive it.

Krishna divides the mental traits and whirlpools or thought processes into two groups - Daivi-sampada and Asuri-sampada. All Sattvic mental traits and processes are under the Daivi-Sampat while the mental processes under the rajasaic and tamasic qualities come under the Asuri-Smapada. Daivi-sampada leads us towards Atma-Jnana or Knowledge of the Self. The Asuri-Sampada mental processes are known to be obstacles on the spiritual path. Everyone in the world falls under one or other of these categories of mental traits. People following the spiritual path to attain liberation must follow the sattvic life and avoid rajasic and tamasic tendencies.

Krisha details the following traits of daivi-sampada:

1. Fearlessness
2. Purity
3. Scriptural Study
4. Charity
5. Sense-control
6. Worship of God
7. Austerity
8. Straightforwardness
9. Non-violence, kindness to all and absence of ill-will
10. Truthfulness
11. Renunciation
12. Calmness and patience
13. Absence of slander
14. Absence of greed
15. Gentleness
16. Modesty
17. Steadfastness and absence of restlessness
18. Strength

Asuri-sampada
1. Vanity
2. Arrogance
3. Pretension
4. Anger

5.   Cruelty
6.   Ignorance
7.   Impurity
8.   Absence of religious discipline
9.   Absence of truthfulness
10.   Absence of faith in God
11.   Endless desire for sense- pleasure
12.   Delusion
13.   False values
14.   Attachment
15.   Greed
16.   Egoism
17.   Slander

The three materialistic mental traits are a major cause of worldly suffering. These traits are desire, anger, and greed. By avoiding these three negative traits and developing a daivi-sampada mindset and attitude, one qualifies for Atma-Jnana and is led on the path to attain liberation soon.

Krishna mentions that Shastras or valid scriptures are the Pramana (valid knowledge) in distinguishing what is right and wrong. One should study the scriptures and follow the teachings accordingly.

The Field and Its Knower; Kshetra Kshetrajna Vibhagha Yoga

BG 16.1-3: Shri Bhagavan said: O offspring of Bharat, these are the pious virtues of those established in the divine nature - fearlessness, purity of mind, steadfastness in spiritual knowledge, charity, control of the senses, performance of sacrifice, study of the sacred scriptures, austerity, and straightforwardness; non-violence, honesty, free from anger, renunciation, peacefulness, free from fault-finding, compassion toward all living beings, absence of greediness, gentleness, modesty, and lack of fickleness; vigour, forgiveness, fortitude, cleanliness, bearing enmity toward none, and absence of vanity.

In these three verses Lord Krishna reveals the Sattvic mental traits known as Daivi-Sampada:

1.   Abhayam - fearlessness
2.   Sattva Sanshuddhih - purity of mind
3.   Jnana-Yoga-Vyavashitih - steadfastness in yoga of self-knowledge
4.   Danam - charity
5.   Damah - sensory discipline
6.   Yajnah - performing sacrificial duties
7.   Swadhyaya - Studying sacred scriptures and introspection or self-study
8.   Tapah - austerity and dedication in Sadhana
9.   Arajavam - straightforwardness
10. Ahimsha - Non-violence, non-injury
11. Satyam- Honesty or truthfulness
12. Akrodhah - free from anger

13. Tyagah - renunciation and giving away that which is not necessary
14. Shantih - peacefulness
15. Apaishunam - free from finding faults
16. Daya bhuteshu - compassion towards all living beings
17. Aloluptvam - free from covetouseness
18. Mardvam - gentleness
19. Hrih - Modesty
20. Achapalam - free from fickleness
21. Tejah - vigour
22. Kshama - forgiveness
23. Dhritih - courage and determination
24. Shaucham - cleanliness and purity
25. Adrohaha - free from enmity
26. Na-ati-manita - absence of arrogance and egoism

BG 16.4: O Parth, the qualities of those who possess a demoniac nature (asuri sampada) are hypocrisy (Dambha), arrogance (darpah), arrogance and pride (abhimana), anger (krodha), cruelty (parushyam), and ignorance (ajnana).

BG 16.5: The divine qualities lead the sadhaka towards liberation (vimokshaya), while the demoniac qualities are the root cause for a continuing fate of bondage. O Arjun, no need to grieve as you were born with righteous virtues.

BG 16.6: There are two kinds of living beings (bhuta-jiva) in this world—those blessed with a divine nature or mental traits (daivi-sampada) and those possessing a demoniac nature or mind set (asuri sampada). I have described the divine qualities in detail, O Arjun. Now listen about the demoniac nature from me.

BG 16.7: Those acquiring a demoniac nature are unable to realise what actions are appropriate (pravrattim) and what are inappropriate (nivrattim). Hence, they do not have purity (saucham), or good conduct (su-achara), or even truthfulness (satyam).

In last few verses Krishna explains that people who have daivi-sampada naturally follow their Dharma, which consists of a virtuous code of conduct which is beneficial to one and all and purifies one's body, mind and heart. While people possessing the asura-sampada have no ability to understand or know what is right and wrong and hence engage in Adharma or non-righteous activities which are degrading or destructive to all and everyone.

BG 16.8: They (asura-sampada) say, "The world is without absolute truth (asatya-jagat), without any foundation of moral order (apratishtham), and there is no Divine or Supreme Self (anishvaram). It has been created without a purpose (a-parasparma) from the conception between the two opposite genders, and has no purpose other than sexual gratification (kama-haitukam)."

BG 16.9: Holding strongly to such views, these misguided souls (nashta-atman), with very little intellect (alpa-buddhiya) and cruel actions (ugra-karmanah), ascend as enemies (ahita) of the world threatening to destroy it (kshaya-jagat).

"As long as you live, enjoy yourself. If drinking ghee gives you pleasure, then do so even if you have to take a debt for the purpose. When the body is cremated, you will cease to exist, and will not come back in the world again (so do not worry of any karmic consequences of your actions)." (Charvaka Darshan Based on Materialistic Fulfilment -Bhautikavad Darshana)

BG 16.10: Embracing (ashritya) greedy and never-ending lust (kamam), full of hypocrisy (dambha), pride and arrogance (maan), the Asura-Sampada-Jiva clings to their false doctrines (mada-anvita). Under this illusion (moha), they are attracted to the impermanent and perform their actions with impure intentions.

BG 16.11: They are consumed in endless anxieties (Aparimaya-chintah) that end with death only (pralaya-antah). Still, they remain occupied in the gratification of desires (kama-upabhoga) and for them accumulation of material wealth is the uppermost purpose of life.

"People suffer with indescribable worries and stress in worldly accomplishments—bringing up children and grandchildren, engaging in business, accumulating wealth and treasures, and acquiring fame. If they show the same level of affection, desire and intention for developing love for Shri Krishna's lotus feet, they will never again have to worry about Yamraj, the lord of death as they will be liberated from the cycle of birth and death." (Sukti Sudhakar)[v3]

BG 16.12: Burdened and captivted by hundreds of desires (asha-pasha), and driven by lust and anger (kama-krodha), they strive to accumulate wealth (artham) by unjust means (anyayenah), all for the gratification of their senses.

The Bhagavatam states: "One is allowed to keep only that which is necessary for one's maintenance and the rest should be given in charity to those who need it. If one accumulates more than one's need, one is a thief in the eyes of the divine, and will be punished for it."

BG 16.13-15: The people with a demoniac nature think, "I have gained so much wealth today, and I shall now fulfil my desires. This is mine, and I shall have even more tomorrow. I have destroyed my enemy, and I shall destroy the others too! I am like God himself, I am the enjoyer, I am mighty, and I am joyful. I am wealthy and I have highly positioned relatives. No one else is equal to me! I shall perform ritualistic sacrifices (yajna); I shall give to charities (dana); I shall rejoice (bhogah)." In this way, they are deluded by ignorance.

The Sukti Sudhakar details the following types of people:

Tyagi or Vairagi – One who sacrifices their self-interest for the welfare of others. (Swarth Parityage)

Manava or Manushya – one who engages in the welfare of themselves and others without harming themselves or others. (Swarth Bandhane)

Karma-Phala-Bhogi or Samasari – these have the demonic mindset to fulfil their desires and wouldn't mind if it harms others to fulfil their own needs. (swarthya-nighante)

Dushta-Prakriti – these kind of people find joy in harming others.

This verse is revealing how I-ness, Egoism and negative pride become obstacles on the path of spirituality.

Tao Te Ching states: "Instead of trying to be the mountain, be the valley of the Universe."

Jesus also mentions that: "When you are invited, go and sit in the lowest place so that when the host comes, he may say to you, friend, move up higher. For everyone who exalts himself will be humbled, and everyone who humbles himself will be exalted."

Saint Kabir states: "Water does not flow upward; it naturally flows downward. Those who are humble and modest drink God's grace in their heart, while those who are caught in pride and arrogance remain thirsty."

ūñche pānī na tike, nīche hī thaharāye
nīchā hoya so bhari pī, ūñchā pyāsā jāya !

BG 16.16: Obsessed and controlled astray (vibhrante) by such conceptions, enclosed in a mesh of delusion, and addicted to the enjoyment of sensory pleasures, they descend to the darkest hell (narke-patani).

Ramayan mentions that "Karma or actions are important in this world. Whatever actions people perform, they receive the relative fruits. Hence one will always face the consequences of Karma."

The Bible states: "Be certain your sin will find you out."
"Those who follow their Karma under the sattvic nature attain the higher levels of existence; those who act under the rājasic nature remain in the middle regions; and those who act under the qualities of tāmasic nature are sloping downward to the lower levels of existence." (Garud Purāna)

BG 16.17: Such self-induleged (atma-sambhavitah) and stubborn people (stabdha), full of pride and arrogant in their wealth (dhana-maan-mada), perform sacrifices for showing of wealth in name only (dambhena-naam-yajna), with no regard to the guidelines of the scriptures.

Mahabharat states that: "If we publicise a good deed we have done, its excellence decreases; if we keep it secret, its merit multiplies."

BG 16.18: Blinded by egotism (ahamkara), strength (balam), arrogance (darpam), desire (vaasana), and anger (krodha), the demonic people (abhyasika) abuse the presence of the divine within their own body and in the bodies of others.

BG 16.19-20: These cruel (krura) and hateful (dushtah) people, the awful and malicious of humankind (nara-adhaman), I constantly launch into the wombs of those with similar demoniac natures in the cycle of rebirth in the material world (Bhuta-Jagat). These ignorant souls (ajnana-bhuta-jiva) take birth again and again in demoniac wombs (asura-garbha). Failing to attain me, O Arjun, they gradually sink to the most dreadful type of existence.

BG 16.21: These types of activities (tri-vidham) leading one to the hell (narkam) of self-destruction (nashanam) for the soul—lust (kaam), anger (krodha), and greed (lobha). So one should always abandon these three.

BG 16.22: Those who remain free from those three gates to darkness (tamah-dwara) endeavour for the welfare of their soul (atma-shreya), and thereby attain the supreme goal.

BG 16.23: Those who act under the urge of desire (kam-kartah), discarding the teachings or methods of the scriptures (shastra-vidhim), they never attain perfection (siddhim), or happiness (sukha), or the supreme goal (param-gati) in life.

BG 16.24: Therefore, know and have faith in authority in the scriptures in determining what should be done (karya) and what should not be done (akarya). Understand the scriptural guidelines, activities to be done and the teachings, and then perform your actions in this world appropriately.

The Manu Smriti states: "The authenticity of any spiritual principle of the past, present, or future, must be established on the basis of the Vedas."

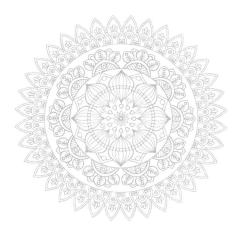

Chapter 17
The Threefold Path;
Shraddhatraya Vibhaga Yoga

In the previous chapter Lord Krishna concluded that we should follow the teachings of the Shastras or scriptures as the Pramana (valid knowledge) to determine what is right and what is wrong to do in life. This chapter begins with Arjuna asking a question:- "To what category of Tri-Gunas (Sattva, Rajas, or Tamas) a person belongs to when he or she is following the path of worship and devotion without scriptural knowledge?"

Krishna mentions that even people performing worship or following the path of devotion may belong to any of the Gunas depending on their temperament, intention and desires.

These people follow the path of devotion or worship by seeing others performing them and they gradually develop faith according to their own character. The person who follows the path of devotion and worship based on scriptural teachings will have the sattvic faith by nature.

Our faith or Sraddha is of three types based on the goal or object of the worship. Krishna mentions that the nature of worship also varies according to the nature of faith. The three types of faith are:

Sattvic Shraddha - pure faith in the divine, free of selfish desires
Rajasic Shraddha- faith in the divine for the sake of fruits and accomplishments
Tamasic Shraddha- faith that involves torturous and toxic practices to gain powers to fulfil material desires

Krishna further details that the Yajnas, Tapas and Daan or Charity can be differentiated in three categories based on the Gunas. A Sadhaka or seeker needs to choose the sattvic type (daivi samada) and avoid rajasic and tamasic types (asuri-sampada).

Lord Krishna concludes this chapter by describing the beauty and significance of the mantra "om tat sat". This sacred mantra originated from the mouth of Brahma at the very beginning of creation and is traditionally chanted in Sanatan Dharma during spiritual activities like Yajna, Tapas and Daana. The word 'sat' means truth, reality, existence, goodness, and virtue. Om is the primordial sound of the divine and the foundation of creation. This mantra translates as "the divine Om is the ultimate reality". This mantra purifies our mind, heart and soul and leads us to divine realisation or Atma-Jnana and Brahma-Jnana.

Finally Krishna mentions that "without Shraddha or faith, all spiritual activities become fruitless or 'asat'."

Gunas	Sattvic	Rajasic	Tamasic
Shraddha or faith	Worship of Gods	Worship of Yakshas and Rakshasas	Worship of spirits and ghosts
Vaasana or desire	Divine Realisation	Worldly Fruits	Power and Sensory Fulfilment
Ahara	Delicious food, which brings longevity, health, strength, and happiness.	excessively bitter, sour, salty, hot, pungent and which causes pain	improperly cooked, without nutrition, putrid, stale, left over, and impure
Yajna	Followed sincerely according to scriptures free from worldly desires	Done for sake of worldly fruits and showing off	Done without scriptural rules, faith, mantra, dakshina or food-offerings
Daanam or charity	sincerely given to a deserving person at the proper time and place without expecting any return	reluctantly given for the sake of return and result	given without respect to an undeserving person at an improper time and place

The Threefold Path; Shraddhatraya Vibhaga Yoga

BG 17.1: Arjun asked: O Krishna, where do they stand in their faith in sattva, rajas and tamas who disregard the teachings of the scriptures (shastra vidhim), but still worship (yajante) with faith?

BG 17.2: Shri Bhagawan said: Every human being (dehinam) is born with innate faith (shraddha), which can be of three kinds—sattvic, rajasic, or tamasic. Now hear about these from me.

BG 17.3: The faith of all human beings (sarva-purusha) follows the nature of their minds (sattva-anurupa). All people enjoy faith, what and who they are depends on the nature of their faith (yata-shradhaya).

BG 17.4: Those with the sattvic guna (quality or nature of goodness) worship the heavenly gods; those with the rajasic guna (quality or nature of passion) worship the Yakshas and Rakshasas; those with the tamsic guna (nature or quality of ignorance) worship ghosts and spirits (preta-bhuta-ganani).

BG 17.5-6: Some people perform severe austerities (ghora-tapah) which are not as per the scriptures (ashastra-vidhitam), motivated by hypocrisy (dambha) and egoism (ahamkara). Urged by desire (kaam) and attachment (raga), they torture parts of their own body (sharira-anga-adi) and also dwell in the body believing this is the Supreme Self. These senseless people are known to be of demonic nature or resolve (asura-nishchayam)

BG 17.7: A person also prefers food (ahara) according to their natures (tri-vidha or tri-gunas). Similarly, it is also true for the sacrifice (yajna), austerity (tapas), and charity (daan) they are inclined towards. Further hear about the distinctions from me.

According to the Chhandogya Upanishad "the coarsest part of the food we eat passes out as faeces; the subtler part becomes flesh; and the subtlest part becomes the mind" (6.5.1).

The Chhandogya Upanishad futher states: ahara shuddhau sattva shuddhih (7.26.2) "By eating pure food, the mind becomes pure."

BG 17.8: A sattvic person under the quality of goodness prefers foods that promote the life span (ayuh-sattva), and increase virtue, strength (bala), health (swasthya), happiness (sukham), and satisfaction (santusthi). Such foods are juicy (rasayah), succulent (snigdha), nourishing (sthirah), and naturally tasteful to the soul (hridaya).

BG 17.9: Persons under the Rajas Guna are attracted to foods that are too bitter (ati-katu), too sour (ati-amla), salty (lavana), very hot (ati-lavana), pungent (tikshna), dry (ruksha), and very spicy. Such foods generate pain (dukha), grief (shoka), and disease (Amaya- disease caused due to toxic food).

BG 17.10: Persons under active Tamas Guna like foods (bhojanam) that are overcooked, stale (yata-yaman), decomposed (puti), polluted (parushytam), tasteless (gata-rasam) and impure (amedhyama).

According to the Ayurvedic Diet, any food that is more than 3 hours (yam) old, becomes tamasic in quality. Also stale, long term stored food, all forms of meat products are classified as tamasic food and they not only cause toxicity in our body but also affect our mindset and karma.

BG 17.11: A Sattvic Yajna or Sacrifice is performed according to the scriptural teachings and guidelines (shastra-vidhih) without expecting the fruits of it (aphala-akanksha), with the firm belief of the mind that it is a subject of duty (dharma-vishaya).

A Yajna or Spiritual ritual should be performed:

❏ Aphala-akankshibhih - without expectation of any fruit or reward.
❏ Vidhi drishtah - according to the teachings, proceedings and guidelines of the Vedic scriptures
❏ Yashtavyam evaiti - should be performed only for the sake of worship of the Divine

BG 17.12: O best of the Bharatas, know that Yajna, which is performed for worldly fruits (artha-phalam), or with hypocritical goals (dambha-phalam), is to be classified as Rajasic Yajna.

BG 17.13: Yajna lacking of faith (shraddha-vrihitam) and in opposition to the teachings and methods of the scriptures (shastra-vidhi-hinam), without offering of food (prashadam), without chanting of the mantras (mantra-hinam), and with no donation made (adakshinam), is to be considered as Tamasic Yajna.

BG 17.14: Worship of the Supreme Divine done with the observance (niyamas) of cleanliness (shaucha), simplicity (arjavam), non-violence (ahimsha), celibacy and free from worldly desires (Brahmachariya) by the Brahmins, the spiritual master (Guru), the wise (Prajna), and the elders is known as the Sharira Tapah or austerity of body.

BG 17.15: Words (vakyam) that do not cause distress (anudvega karam), are truthful (satya), inoffensive and beneficial (Priya-hitam), as well as the regular recitation of the Vedic scriptures (swadhyaya-abhyasam)—these are classified as the austerity of speech (vaan-mayam-tapas).

satyam bruyat priyam bruyan na bruyat satyam apriyam priyam cha nanritam bruyat esha dharmah sanatanah (Manu Smriti 4.138)

"Speak the truth. Speak the truth in a pleasing manner to others. Do not speak the truth in a harmful manner to others. Do not speak untruth, though it may be pleasant. This is the eternal path of morality and dharma (santan dharma)."

BG 17.16: Tranquillity of mind (manas-prasadam), gentleness (saumyatvam), silence (mauna), self-control (atma-vinigraha), and purity of desires and goals (bhava-sanshuddhi) are known to be the Tapah-Mansa or austerity of mind.

Sakshi Sadhana (Witnessing Awareness): -

"Witness your thoughts, before they become words and facts. Witness your words, before they become choices, actions and reactions. Witness your choices, actions, and reactions before they become habits. Witness your habits, before they become character. Witness your character, before it becomes your fate."

BG 17.17: When a devoted person (shraddhaya) with enthusiastic faith practices these three-fold austerities (tri-vidha-tapah) without desiring for worldly fruits (aphala-akankshibhih), their Tapas or austerity is known to be sattvic or pure in nature.

BG 17.18: Austerity (tapas) that is performed for showiness (dambha) or the sake of fruits (phala), honour (pratistha), respect (maan), and adoration is known to be Rajasic Tapas or the mode of passion. Fruits of this kind of tapas are transitory and short-lived.

BG 17.19: (Mudha-Grahena-Tapah) Austerity that is performed with confused beliefs, and which involves torturing the self or harming others (atma-pidya), is classified as Tamasic Tapas.

BG 17.20: Charity (Daanam) given to a worthy person (daatavyam) purely because it is right to give, without expecting anything in return from that person, at the proper time (kaala) and in the proper place (desha), is known to be the Sattvic Daan.

The Bhavishya Puran states: "In the Kaliyuga, charity is the means for purification."

Ramayana also mentions that "Dharma has four basic principles, amongst them the most important one in Kaliyuga is charity by whatever means possible."

BG 17.21: But charity given with unwillingness, with the hope of a return (prati-upakara-astham) or in expectation of a fruit or reward (phalam udhishya), is described as Rajasic Daan.

BG 17.22: The charity which is given at the wrong place (adesha), at the wrong time (akaale) and to unworthy persons (apatribhya), without showing respect (asat-kirtam), or with disapproval (avajnatam), is known to be Tamasic Daana.

BG 17.23: The mantra "Om Tat Sat" has been acknowledged as symbolic representation (nirdesha) of the Supreme Absolute

Truth (Brahman), from the beginning of creation. From this arise the priests (Brahamins), scriptures (Shastras), and sacrifice (Yajna).

BG 17.24: Therefore, when performing Yajna, offering charity, or undertaking Tapas, speakers of the Vedas (Brahma-vadinam) always begin by chanting or uttering the Mantra "Om" according to the recommendations of Vedic teachings.

BG 17.25: Persons who are free from desires for fruits (anabhisandhaya-phalam), but seek to be free from material attachments (moksha-kankabhih), utter the mantra "Tat" along with acts of tapas, yajna and daan.

BG 17.26-27: The mantra "Sat" means eternal truth or reality and goodness. O Arjun, it is also used to describe an auspicious action (prashaste karmani). Being established in the performance of Yajna, Tapas and Daan, is also described by the sabda or word "Sat." And so any act for such purposes is known to be "Sat."

Sankalpa Sadhana:

Sat-Bhave – all that has manifested belongs to eternal reality and goodness or purity.
Sadhu-Bhave – All that I need is pure and auspicious intensions.
Sat-Prashaste Karmani – I perform all my actions with pure intentions.
Ahama-Sat-Sthite – I am well established in Truth, Reality or Essence of Life.
Sat-Sabda-Vachani – I speak what is absolute truth and sweet and fruitful for all beings.

Sat-artham-Bhava – I see the divine reality in all.

BG 17.28: O Partha, whatever acts of Yajna or Tapas are done without faith, are termed as "Asat." They are useless both in this world and the next.

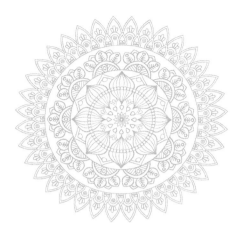

Chapter 18
Liberation Through Renunciation;
Moksha Sanyasa Yoga

In this chapter Arjuna requests that Krishna explain to him the nature and difference between Sanyasa and Tyaga.

Krishna begins his teachings by emphasising the importance of important Dharma practices (nitya-karma) like Yajna, Daan, and Tapas. We should never give up on these virtuous human acts. These selfless acts will help a Sadhaka to purify his mind, heart, karma and samskaras. Krishna mentions that a person who has attained absolute purity may not need to perform these nitya-karmas. Krishna further describes Sanyasa of three types - tamasic, rajasic, and sattvic.

A sattvic renunciation according to Lord Krishna is nothing other than Karma Yoga. A Karma Yogic renounces the fruits of his or her actions (niskama-karma). By means of karma yoga, he attains Atma-Jnana or self-knowledge. A sannyasi or karma yogi is free from the consequences of good, evil or a mix of both.

Further Lord Krishna reveals the essence of Jnana Yoga. In every Karma, five factors are always involved. These are:- the body (deha), Prana, the mind (manas) with senses (indriyas), the ego (ahamkara) and the governing divinity (Jiva and Prakriti) of all these. All the good and evil actions are performed by means of these five factors. The Purusha or Self is never involved in any of the Karmic actions and/ or choices and their consequences. But due to our ignorance, we identify our true self with the above five factors and mistake the Self as the doer (karta). A Jnani or wiseman, free from the Asmita or 'I-ism' or Ahamkara is also free from all the karmas, even though he is the instrument of all the activities performed by means of the five factors. The Purusha is neither a doer (akarta), nor a consumer (a-bhokta).

Krishna explains the six necessary factors in any of our actions, interactions and behavioural patterns (vyavahara). These are:

Jnata - the Knower
Jnana - the knowledge
Jneya - the known
Karta - the doer
Karma - the action
Karma Yantra- the instrument of action

Our Jnana, Karma and Karta are further classified in three divisions based on the three gunas. Our Buddhi or intellect also has the three categories based on the gunas. Also our

Sukha or happiness has three types according to the gunas. Krishna mentions that nothing in this world of creation is free from the three gunas.

Guna	Sattva	Rajas	Tamas
Sanyasa / renunciation	Renunciation of the fruits of nityakarmas	Renunciation of nityakarmas due to fear of straining the body	Renunciation of nityakarmas due to the ignorance of their value
Jnanam / Knowledge	Advaita – sees the undivided eternal Self in and all beings	Sees the one distinct from everything else	Sees the body as the ultimate self
Karma / Action	Dharma or duties performed without expectation of fruits	Karma done out of ego and desire for the fruits	Kukarma- Indiscriminate action done without considering the consequences
Karta / Doer	detached, perseverant, enthusiastic, humble, and equanimity in success and failure.	attached, greedy, harmful, and subject to excitement and depression	undisciplined, uncultured, arrogant, harmful, dull and procrastinating
Buddhi / Intellect	knows dharma and adharma, right and wrong as well as the bondage and liberation	improperly knows dharma and adharma, as well as right and wrong	knows dharma and adharma, as well as right and wrong irrationally
Dhriti / The Will	one sustains the functions of all body organs on the spiritual path and which is made steadfast through yoga	Follows dharma, artha and karma, for their fruits	caught up in sleep, fear, grief and indulgence
Sukham / Happiness	Ananda born of Self-Knowledge or Atma-Jnana	Born of contact between sense organs and objects or fruits	born of laziness and negligence.

The duties or Dharma of the four Varnas (classes of people - which are Brahmanas, Kshatriyas, Vaisyas, and Sudras) are described in **scriptures according to their nature. Karma Yoga** is to perform one's own dharma as an offering to the Divine. This prepares the mind to be fit for Atma-Jnana. According to Krishna Swadharma (skills and abilities we are blessed with to perform particular tasks or actions) are most important to be performed by each individual. We need to perform our dharma for sake of purity, social harmony and learning lessons. Not doing our duties will only lead us to confusion and suffering. A pure sadhaka, detached from all the worldly objects and fruits of all the actions and self-controlled (atma-sanyami) will soon attain liberation through jnana-yoga.

Krishna further gives a brief teaching on meditation or nidhi-dhyasanam to receive necessary knowledge through listening and thinking (shravanam, mananam). Begin by choosing a comfortable and steady position for the body. Free from disturbing thoughts arising from desires, anger etc., one should remain in a secluded place. By being firm in the divine nature of his own Brahma, he attains freedom from grief and desire. He remains the same or equanimous towards all beings and enjoys the highest devotion to the Supreme Self or Iswara. By knowing the true nature of Parmatman, one becomes one with the Divine. This is merely realisation of the advaita (non-duality) nature of Purusha and Parmatman.

Again, Krishna emphasises the importance of Karma yoga and Bhakti-Karma Yoga, where we surrender or offer all our actions to the divine purpose. By remembering the divine in each of our thoughts, actions and feelings, ultimately he becomes one with the Divine.

If one tries to escape the duty assigned to him based on his nature, it will be harmful, unproductive and vain. A devotee should surrender his heart, actions and all to the supreme

Divine, who is the controller of all, to attain absolute bliss (ati-ananda) and supreme peace (Ananta-shanti).

Krishna concludes that Arjuna should now make his own choice and do what he wishes to do. Krishna tells him that he has revealed many ways to attain to liberation. He repeats again, "Fix your mind on Me. Be My devotee. Be My worshiper. Surrender to Me. You shall reach Me alone. Truly I promise to you. You are dear to Me. Having renounced all actions, seek Me, the nondual, as your shelter. I shall liberate you from all sins. Do not grieve"

Krishna mentions that these teachings are not for the one who has no faith, discipline, devotion and desire to know. One who learns, understands and follows these practices in life, will certainly attain the Supreme Divine. Even if we listen to these teachings with faith, we will attain higher abodes or worlds.

Finally Krishna asks Arjuna if he is satisfied with the teachings and whether his delusion is gone. Arjuna expresses his gratitude, acknowledges the teachings and promises to follow these divine teachings.

The Bhagavad Gita is concluded by Sanjaya addressing Dhratarashtra about how blessed he was to be able to listen to this glorious and divine dialogue between Lord Krishna and Arjuna. He remembers all the teachings and the cosmic vision of Krishna.

Sanjay concludes with his statement, "where there is Krishna, the lord of yoga, and where there is Arjuna, the master of the bow, there will be eternal wealth, victory, prosperity and justice".

Liberation Through Renunciation; Moksha Sanyasa Yoga

BG 18.1: Arjun said: O mighty-armed Krishna, I wish to (icchami) understand the nature of sannyas (total renunciation) and tyag (renunciation of the possessions or sensory objects). O Hrishikesh, I also wish to know the difference between the two, O Keshinisudan.

BG 18.2: The Supreme Divine said: Giving up (nyasam) of actions (karma) inspired by desire (kamyamam) is what the wise understand as sannyas. Renouncing the fruits of all actions (sarva-karma-phala) is declared to be tyaga by learned ones.

BG 18.3: Some learned people (manishinah) state firmly that all kinds of actions should be given up as evil, while others mention that acts of Yajna, Daan and Tapas (sacrifice, charity, and penance) should never be abandoned.

BG 18.4: O tiger (vyagraha) amongst the men, in my conclusion renunciation has been known to be of three kinds (tri-vidha).

BG 18.5: Actions based upon sacrifice, charity, and penance should never be abandoned; they must certainly be performed. Indeed, acts of Yajna, Daan and Tapas are purifying (pavanani) even for those who are wise.

BG 18.6: O Arjun, these activities must be performed free from attachment (sangam-tyaga) and without the desiring for fruits (phala-tyaga). This is my definite (nischitam) and supreme verdict (uttamam).

BG 18.7: Prearranged duties by birth (niyatasya) should never be renounced. Such deluded (mohat) renunciation is known to be in the tamasic guna.

BG 18.8: To give up the assigned duties because they are difficult (klesha) or cause physical discomfort (deha-dukham) is renunciation in the rajasic guna. Such renunciation is never fruitful or inspirational.

BG 18.9: When Karma or actions are taken as a Dharma or duty (karma niyate- obligatory actions), Arjun, and one renounces attachment to any fruit (phala-mukti), it is considered renunciation in the sattvic guna.

BG 18.10: Those who do not avoid displeasing work (akushalam karma) as well as do not seek work because it is pleasant (kushale) are persons of true renunciation (chinne-Sanyasa). They are established in the sattva guna or the quality of goodness.

BG 18.11: For the living being (deha-bhrita), it is impossible to renounce the activities completely. But those who renounce the fruits of their actions are known to be truly renounced (karma-phala-tyagi).

BG 18.12: The three-fold fruits (tri-vidham-phala) of actions— pleasant (ishtam), unpleasant (anishtam), and mixed (mishram)—accumulate even after death to those who are attached to the fruits (atyaginam). But, for those who renounce the fruits of their actions, there are no such results in the here or hereafter.

- Ishtam, or pleasant experiences in the higher states (Swarga-Lokah)
- Anishtam, or unpleasant experiences in the lower fields of consciousness (Narka-Lokah)
- Mishram, or mixed experiences in the human form on the earth planet (Bhu-lokah)

BG 18.13: O Arjun, now listen to me about the five factors (pancha-karnani) that have been mentioned for the execution of all actions in the teachings of Sankhya, which also reveals how to stop the reactions of karmas.

BG 18.14: The body (adhisthanam), the doer (karta), the sense organs with the mind (indriyas), the many kinds of efforts (vividha-chesta), and Divine Wisdom (daivyam)—these are the five factors of action.

Prashna Upanishad mentions that "It is the soul that sees, touches, hears, feels, tastes, thinks, and comprehends. Thus, the soul is to be considered both—the knower and the doer of actions."

The Brahma Sūtra also states that, "It is truly the soul that is the knower."

The Brahma Sūtra further states that, "The soul is the doer of actions, and this is confirmed by the scriptures."

Niti Shastra mentions that, "With appropriate effort, even poor destiny can be transformed into good fortune; and, "Without appropriate effort, even good destiny can be altered into misfortune."

BG 18.15-16: These five are the instrumental factors for whatever action is performed, whether appropriate (nyayayam) or inappropriate (viparitam), with body, speech, or mind (sharia-vak-manobhi). Those who do not know this, they see the soul as the only doer. With their impure intellects (akrita-bhuddhi) they cannot see things as they are.

The Kenopanishad states:

"Brahma cannot be described by the words and speech. By its inspiration, the words get the power to speak."

"Brahma cannot be understood by the mind and intellect. By its power, the mind and intellect get the power to understand."

"Brahma cannot be seen with the eyes. By its inspiration, the eyes see."

"Brahma cannot be heard with the ears. By its power, the ears hear."

"Brahma cannot be energised by the prana vayus. By its inspiration, the prana vayus function."

BG 18.17: Those who are free from the Ahamkara (I-ism, or Ego) of being the doer (karta bhava), and whose intellect is unattached, though they may kill living beings, they neither kill nor are they bound by actions.

BG 18.18: Knowledge (jnana), the object of knowledge (jneya), and the knower (parijnata)—these are the three factors that stimulate action. The instrument of action (karanam), the act (karma), and the doer (karta)—these are the three components of action (karma sangraha).

Jnana triputi: - jnana (knowledge), jneya (the object of knowledge), and jnata (the knower) together are called the triad of knowledge.
Karm triputi (triad of action):- includes the karta (doer), karan (the instrument of action), and karma (the act).

BG 18.19: Jnana, karma, and the Karta are announced to be of three kinds in the Sankhya philosophy, distinguished according to the three Gunas of Prakriti. Now I will explain their differences to you.

BG 18.20: A person that realises and sees the all-pervading eternal reality within all living beings has knowledge in the Sattva Guna.

Shrimad Bhagavad mentions that, "Knowers of the truth have affirmed that there is only one entity in existence, without a second."

Four Qualities of Divine Consciousness:

1. Sajatiya bhed shunya - He is one with all similar entities like Krishna, Rama, Shiva, Vishnu etc.

2. Vijatiya bhed shunya - He is one with all different beings due to the divine maya.

3. Swagat bhed shunya - The various parts of his body are non-different from him

The Brahma Samhita states: "With every limb of his body, God can see, hear, talk, smell, eat, and think."

4. Swayam siddha - He is perfect on his own and doesn't need the support of other entities.

BG 18.21: The one with the knowledge under the mode of Rajasic Guna sees the difference in each living being in different bodies and sees them divided or unconnected.

BG 18.22: That knowledge is known to be in the mode of tamasic guna where one is occupied in a fragmental concept as if it includes the whole, and which is neither grounded in reason (ahaitukam) nor based on the truth (atattva-artha).

BG 18.23: Karma that is in harmony with the scriptures, which is free from raga and dvesha (attachment and aversion), and which is performed without the desire for fruits, is in the mode of the sattva guna.

Mahabharat mentions that, "We should not behave with others in a way we don't like others to behave with us. We should always verify that our behaviour is in harmony with the scriptures."

BG 18.24: Action that is driven by selfish desire (kama-ipsuna), enacted with pride (ahamkaren), and very stressful, is known to be rajasic in nature.

BG 18.25: The Karma that is performed out of delusion (moha), without thought to one's own abilities, ignoring the consequences, loss and harm to others is known to be tamasic in nature.

BG 18.26: The Karta or doer is said to be in the nature of sattva, when he is free from egoism (ahamkara), and attachment (mukta sanga), brilliant with enthusiasm or zeal (utaha) and determination (dhriti), and maintains equanimity in success and failure (samanvita-siddhi-asiddhaye).

BG 18.27: The Karta is considered in the nature of Rajas when he desires the fruits of the actions (karma-phala-iccha), is jealous (prepsu), violent-natured (himsak), impure (ashuddha), and moved by joy and sorrow (harsha-shoka-anvita).

BG 18.28: A Karta is known to be of tamasic nature when he is undisciplined, ill-mannered, stubborn, deceiving, lazy, hopeless, and procrastinating.

Shrimad Bhagavad also mentions that, "A Karta who is detached is sattvic in nature; the one who is excessively attached to action and its fruits is rajasic; one who is lacking of discrimination is tamasic. But the karta who is renounced to me is transcendental to the three gunas of prakriti."

BG 18.29: O Arjun, now listen about the divisions of intellect (buddhi) and willpower or determination (dhriti), according to the three gunas of prakriti, as I describe them in detail.

BG 18.30: The Buddhi is said to be in the nature of sattva, O Parth, when it understands what is appropriate karma (karya) and what is inappropriate karma (akarya), what is duty (dharma) and what is non-duty (adharma), what is to be feared (bhaya) and what is not to be feared (abhaya), what is binding (bandhaya) and what is liberating (mokshaya).

BG 18.31: The buddhi is known to be in the rajasic prakriti when it is confused between righteousness (dharma) and unrighteousness (adharma), and cannot discriminate between right and wrong conduct (kariyam-akariyam).

BG 18.32: The Buddhi which is shrouded in darkness, imagining adharma to be dharma, and seeing the untruth to be the truth, is said to be tamasic in nature.

BG 18.33: The steadfast will (dhriti) that is developed through Yoga, and which sustains the activities of the mind, the prana vayus, and the senses (indriyas), is said to be sattvic in nature.

BG 18.34: The firm willpower by which one holds duty (dharma), pleasures (sukham), and wealth (artham), out of attachment and desire for fruit (phala-iccha), is rajasic dhriti in nature.

BG 18.35: That thoughtless determination (dhrumedha) or willpower is known to be tamasic in nature, in which one does not give up dreaming (swapnam), fearing (Bhaya), grieving (shoka), despair (vishadam), and conceit (madam).

BG 18.36: And now listen, O Arjun, there are three kinds of happiness (sukham) in which the living being rejoices (ramate), and can even lead to the end of all suffering (dukkha-antam).

BG 18.37: That which seems like poison (visham) at first, but tastes like nectar (amrita) in the end, is said to be happiness of the sattvic nature. It is produced by the pure intellect (prashad-jam) that is situated in self-knowledge (atma buddhi).

Kathopanishad states that, "There are two paths—one is the 'beneficial in evolution' and the other is the 'pleasant'. These two leads one to very different ends. The pleasant is enjoyable in the beginning, but it ends in suffering. The ignorant follow the path of pleasure and suffer at the end. But the wise choose the beneficial path, which may seem to be painful in beginning, but finally attain absolute bliss or happiness."

BG 18.38: Happiness is mentioned to be rajasic in nature when it is resulting from the contact (sanyogat) of the senses (indiya) with their objects (visayanam). Such happiness is like nectar in the beginning but results in suffering at the end.

BG 18.39: That happiness which hinders the true nature of the self from beginning to end, and which is resulting from sleep (nidra), laziness (alasya), and negligence (pramada), is said to be the tamsic sukham in nature.

BG 18.40: No living being on earth or the higher heavenly abodes in this material world is free from the authority of these three gunas of the Prakriti.

Swatashwar Upanishad states that, "Prakriti has three colours—white, red, and black, i.e. it has three modes—sattva, rajas and tamas. It is the mother-like womb of the countless living beings within the universe. It is brought into existence and supported by the one unborn eternal all-pervading Supreme Consciousness, who is all-knowing Parmatman. Divine, itself is however free and beyond its own created Prakriti. He independently enjoys the pleasure of his transcendental nature. But the living being or Jiva enjoys enough pleasure within his own body by means of senses and mind and thus becomes bound."

BG 18.41: The duties (karmani) of the Brahmins, Kshatriyas, Vaishyas, and Shudras are distributed according to their qualities, in accordance with their gunas.

BG 18.42: Tranquillity (sham), restraint (dam), austerity (tapas), purity (shaucha), patience (kshati), integrity (arjavam), knowledge (jnana), wisdom (viveka), and belief (shraddha) are the inherent qualities of a Brahmins Dharma.

BG 18.43: Valour (shauryam), strength (balam), determination (dhriti), skill in artillery (yuddha-dakshe), never to flee from battle (apalayanam), large-heartedness in charity (daanam vishal hridaye), and leadership abilities (ishwara), these are the natural qualities (shwa-bhavaja) of Kshatriyas dharma.

BG 18.44: Agriculture (krishi), dairy farming (gau rakshya), and commerce (vanijyam) are the natural karma for those with the qualities of Vaishyas. Serving others is the natural duty (nihit-karma) for those with the inborn qualities (shwa-bhavaja) of Shudras.

BG 18.45: By performing their karmas, born of their innate qualities (prakriti-gunah), human beings (narah) can attain perfection (siddhih). Now hear from me how one can attain perfection by performing one's prearranged duties (swa-karma also known as swa-dharma).

BG 18.46: By performing one's natural duties (swa-karmani), one worships the All-pervading Divine from whom all living beings (bhutanam) have come into existence. By such performance of Karma, a person easily attains perfection.

BG 18.47: It is better (shreyam) to follow one's own dharma, even if done imperfectly (vigunah), than to follow another's dharma (par-dharma), even though perfectly (su-anusthita). By performing one's innate duties (swa-svabhava-karmani), a person does not earn sin.

Srimada Bhagavad states, "We must keep following our dharma and perform Karmas as long as we have not mastered the Bhakti through hearing, chanting, and meditating on the Supreme Divine Krishna."

BG 18.48: One should not abandon (na-tyajate) duties born of one's nature (saha-jam-karma), even if one sees faults (dosham) in them, O son of Kunti. Indeed, all undertakings (sarva-arambha) are disguised (avrita) by some evil, as fire is covered by smoke (angi-dhumena).

BG 18.49: Those who have intellect without any attachment (asakta-buddhi) from all and everything (sarvatha), who have mastered the mind (jita-atma), and are free from desires (niskam-bhava) by the practice of renunciation (Sanyasa-abhyasa), attain the highest perfection of freedom from action (parmam-naishya-karma-siddhim).

BG 18.50: O Arjuna, now in brief hear from, I shall now reveal how one, who has attained perfection (siddhim-praptah), can also attain Brahman by being firmly established (nistha) in transcendental knowledge (para-jnanasya or para-vidya).

BG 18.51-53: One attains fitness (adhikara) to attain Brahman when he or she possesses a purified intellect (parishudha-buddhi) and firmly contains the senses (indriya-jaya), transcending sound and other objects of the senses (shabda-adin-vishayan-tyaktva), mastering freedom from attraction and aversion (raga-dvesha-mukti). Such a person enjoys solitude (vivikta-sevi), eats lightly (laghu-ashi), controls the body, mind, and speech (yata-deha, vac, manasa), is ever absorbed in meditation (dhyana-yoga-parah), and practices detachment (vairagyam). Free (mukta) from egotism (ahamkara), violence (himsha), arrogance (darpam), desire (kaam), possessiveness of property (nirmamah), and selfishness and accumulation (parigraham), such a person, established in tranquillity (shantah), is appropriately suitable for realisation or oneness with Brahman (Brahma-Bhuyaye-Kalpate).

BG 18.54: One situated in the Absolute Brahma (Brahma-Bhuta) realisation attains serenity of mind (Prasanna-atma), remains free of grieving and desiring (shoka-kaam-mukti). Remaining in equanimity towards all living beings (bhutesu), such a Yogi attains supreme devotion (param-bhakti) unto me.

BG 18.55: Only by loving devotion (bhaktya) to me, one comes to know (abhijanati) who I am in truth (mama-tattvani). Then, by knowing me (jnantva), my devotee enters into full consciousness of me.

BG 18.56: My devotees (mama-bhakta), performing all kinds of actions (sarva-karmani), take full refuge in me (vyapa-shriya). By my grace (prasadat), they attain the eternal and never-ending abode (avapnoti-shasvatam-avyayayam-padam).

BG 18.57: Dedicate your every karma to me (sarva-karmani-Sanyasa), keeping me as your supreme goal (ma-parah). Following the Buddhi-Yoga (Yoga path to keep the intellect absorbed in the divine), always keep your consciousness absorbed in Me.

BG 18.58: By always remembering Me (mata-chitta), with my grace you will overcome all obstacles (durgani) and difficulties. But if, due to pride (ahamkara), you do not listen to my advice, you will perish (vinakshyashi).

BG 18.59: If you think, "I shall not fight" due to your mental misconceptions (mithya-eshah-manas), your decision will be in worthless. Your own Kshatriya nature will require you to fight.

BG 18.60: O Arjun, those Karmas which out of delusion (moha) you do not wish to perform, you will be driven to do by your own true nature, born of your own prakriti (swabhava-jena).

Here Krishna simply states that "Due to our sanskaras of past lives, we are born with an innate nature. Our inborn qualities will compel us to follow a certain path."

BG 18.61: The Supreme Consciousness resides in the hearts of all living beings (bhuta-jiva), O Arjun. According to their karmas, He plants seeds of journeys (bhramaayam) of the souls, who are seated on a machine (yantra-arudhani) made of the material energy (mayayi).

BG 18.62: Surrender absolutely (shranam-gaccha) unto Him wholeheartedly (sarva-bhave), O Bharat. By His grace, you will attain absolute peace (param-shanti) and the eternal consciousness (shashvatam).

BG 18.63: So, I have revealed (akhyatam) to you this knowledge that is most secret (guhyata) of all secrets. Contemplate (vimrishya) it deeply, and then follow as you wish (swa-icchashi).

Once Lord Rama at the end of his discourse to his pupils reminded all that, "The advice I have given to you is neither incorrect nor coercive. Listen to it carefully, contemplate it, and then do what you wish."

BG 18.64: Hear again my supreme instruction, the most confidential knowledge of all the knowledge (sarva-guhya-tamam-vidya). I am revealing (vakshyami) this for your benefit (hitam) because you are very dear to me (mama-priyam).

BG 18.65: Always think of Me (mat-manah), be devoted to Me (mat-bhakta), worship Me (mat-yaji), and practice gratitude to Me (namaskarum). Doing so, you will certainly attain Me. This is my pledge to you, as you are very dear to Me (mama-priyah).

BG 18.66: Renounce all kinds of dharma (sarva-dharmam) and simply surrender unto me alone. I shall liberate (moksha) you from all sinful outcomes (paapebhya); do not fear.

BG 18.67: These teachings should never be revealed to those who are not austere (a-tapasya) or to those who are not devoted (abhaktya). It should not be spoken to those who are unwilling to listen to spiritual teachings (ashushrushave), and especially not to those who are spiteful (abhyuyayti) of Me.

Padam Purana mentions that "By giving spiritual teachings to those who are faithless and opposed to the divine, we make them become offenders."

BG 18.68: Those, who share these most confidential knowledges (param-guhya-vidyam) amongst my devotees, perform the greatest act of love (param-kritva-prema). They will attain me without a doubt.

BG 18.69: That is the most loving service to Me by any human being (manushyanam); no one else ever on this earth other than them is dearer to me.

BG 18.70: And I declare that those who study this sacred discourse (dharmyam-samvadam) of ours will worship me through the sacrifice of knowledge (jnana-yajnena) in my view.

BG 18.71: Even those who only listen (shruniyat) to this knowledge with faith (shraddhayat) and without envy will be liberated from sins (paap-moksha) and attain the auspicious abodes (subham-lokah) where the pious souls reside (punya-karmanam).

BG 18.72: O Arjun, have you heard me with a focussed mind? Have your ignorance (ajnana) and delusion (Sammoha) been removed?

BG 18.73: Arjun Said: O trustworthy one, by your grace my illusion has been dispersed, and I am well established in knowledge. Now I am free from doubts (gata-sandeha), and I shall act according to your teachings.

BG 18.74: Sanjay said: I have heard this magnificent dialogue between Shree Krishna, the son of Vasudev, and Arjun, the noble-hearted son of Pritha. So delightful is the message that I am experiencing goosebumps (roma-harshanam).

BG 18.75: By the grace of Veda Vyas (Vyasa-Prashadah), I have heard this supreme and most secret Yoga Vidya from the Lord of Yoga (Yogeshwar), Shree Krishna himself.

BG 18.76: As I repeatedly remember (sam-smirtya) this overwhelming (adhbhutam) and magnificent dialogue between the Supreme Lord Shree Krishna and Arjun, O King, I rejoice again and again.

BG 18.77: And remembering that most astonishing and wonderful cosmic form (Vishwa-rupa) of Lord Krishna, great is my amazement (maha-vismaya), and I am thrilled (hrishyami) with joy over and over again.

BG 18.78: Wherever there is Shree Krishna, the Master of all Yoga, and wherever there is Arjuna, the supreme archer, there will also certainly be eternal abundance, victory, prosperity, and righteousness. I am very certain of this.

The Bhagavad Gita is a truly groundbreaking yoga text, not least due to its syncretic approach where the seeker is offered multiple practices to choose from and even blend, according to their own particular strengths and weaknesses. As Swami Chinmayananda noted, this approach was intentional – the Puranic world within which the Gita's author, Vyasa, was writing was one of conflict, different schools of thought competing against each other, each saying their way was the only way. Sadly, we find ourselves in a similar position today, even within some of the many commentaries on the Gita.
But not this one.
Yogachariya Jnandev has succeeded where many have failed, presenting the Gita with its true spirit of unity fully intact. His vast experience within spirituality and life, as a sadhu, a yogachariya, a family man and an academic, lends him a uniquely broadminded perspective. Born out of a series of lessons on the Gita he delivered, this commentary offers an understanding of the text that is accessible, pragmatic and profound.
An essential read for yoga sadhakas everywhere.
Dharmananda
(Dharmananda Yoga & Mindfulness)

||Om tat sat||
||That divine is the only reality||

Leading a life of equanimity or balance that is reflected in my thoughts, actions, and ways of connecting with my inner self and what surrounds me is the summation of my life since I did this course. I feel blessed and feel ready to devour "the nectar of life"; The Bhagwat Gita through a Guru like Yogacharya Jnandev. I have experienced that submission to learning like Arjun and a Guru to teach like Shree Krishna are the key to this experience. Gita knowledge is made accessible by Jnandev as he engages the listener in stories from ancient Indian literature like the Upanishads, Samhitas and Vedas and relates them to modern life making it relevant and applicable. This course is accessible to those who are new to this literature and those who want higher understanding of it; where the Gita suggests prescriptive systems of Yoga about how we can live everyday through Nishkam Karma or fruitless action and moving towards Atma Jnan or self- realisation. Jnandev's discourses shine light on the complex subtleties of life in a simple way that are culturally appropriate and maintain the essence of the Sanskrit language. A course that is accessible, thought provoking, and relevant to the current context of modern life; The Bhagwat Gita Course is an eye- opener in its subtlest form.

Sandhya Saldanha
Sanatan Yoga Teacher and Child & Filial Therapist

Bhagavad Gita Feedback

Yogacharya Jnandev's understanding of the broad teachings of the Bhagavad Gita is truly amazing, I can't really put it into words but he translates it so well. I attended the course online and found it really helpful to be able to attend from my home environment. During each session, Yogacharya Jnandev provided an evaluation of each chapter meaning he could really delve into the depths of this ancient and wonderful scripture. As always, Yogacharya Jnandev was able to explore the many meanings in each chapter and explain them in a way that you could not only understand, but associate the meaning to your own life. A description of the key Sanskrit words were provided at the beginning of each session which made it easier to understand the in depth translation that was then provided. After 6 chapters, a questions and answers session was provided to ensure we had all truly understood the teachings. In particular, one session has remained in my memory. I was dealing with some personal issues and was unsure whether to attend that evening, but I did anyway and it was as if I was meant to be there, the teachings were exactly what I needed to hear. Here are some notes I made on Chapter 14: Our mind creates so many situations - maya illusions - which are exacerbated by the sense organs. Develop the eyes of wisdom, nose of wisdom, ears of wisdom, skin of wisdom, tongue of wisdom, which are all connected to the mind and then help to develop the mind of wisdom jnana...We only experience what we are capable of experiencing and understanding...remove what drags you down, connect in a way that takes you up...disassociate yourself from the negative thought patterns bringing you down and away from your higher self...disconnect with the negativities...connect with the positives.

Sanatan Yoga with Isie
www.yogisie.co.uk

Jnandev is an enthusiastic and wonderful teacher, with a deep understanding of the spiritual scriptures: the Bhagavadgita course I followed with him was wonderful! Jnandev really sets the scene of the great battle of Kurukshetra, explaining the often confusing story and dialogue between Krishna and Arjuna in a step by step way, making it easier to follow and incorporate into our daily lives. With the clear teachings from Jnadev and weekly group discussions I have been able to begin to understand this amazing book, my own nature and perspective. Thank you Jnandev for this inspiring course! Hari om tat Sat

Anita Evans
https://anitaevans.co.uk